To Gabrielle and Linda

Preface

Let us go then, you and I,
When the evening is spread out against the sky
Like a patient etherized upon a table;

T. S. Elliott

Since the term was coined some 22 years ago (Guyatt 1991; Moayyedi 2008), evidence-based medicine, or EBM, has taken center stage in the practice of medicine. Adherence to EBM requires medical practitioners to keep abreast of the results of medical research as reported in the general and specialty journals. At the heart of this research is the science of statistics. It is through statistical techniques that researchers are able to discern the patterns in the data that tell a clinical story worth reporting. Like the astronomer's telescope, statistics uncovers a universe that is invisible to the naked eye. But if you are one of those souls for whom the statistical machinations in the medical literature may as well be cuneiform script, this primer is for you. In it, we invite the reader on a stroll through the landscape of statistical science. We will, moreover, view that landscape while it is, in Elliott's words, "etherized upon a table"—anesthetized, inert, harmless.

This primer is intended for anyone who wishes to have a better grasp of the meaning of statistical techniques as they are used in medical research. This includes physicians, nurses, nurse practitioners, physician's assistants, medical students, residents, or even laypersons who enjoy reading research reports in medicine. The book can also be useful for the physician engaged in medical research who is not also a statistician. With the aid of this primer, that researcher will find it easier to communicate with the statisticians on his or her research team. Our intention is to provide a background in statistics that allows readers to understand the application of statistics in journal articles and other research reports in the medical field. It is not our intention to teach individuals how to perform statistical analyses of data or to be statisticians. We leave that enterprise for the many more voluminous works in medical statistics that are out there. Rather the goal in this work is to provide a reader-friendly introduction to the logic and the tools that underlie statistical science.

In pursuit of this goal we have "cut to the chase" to a considerable degree. We felt that it was important to limit attention to the aspects of statistics that the reader was most likely to encounter on a routine basis. And we believed that it was better to devote more space to a few important topics rather than try to inundate the reader with too many different techniques. Thus, we have omitted extensive coverage of, say, the different ways of graphically displaying data. Other than examples of graphs taken from the medical literature, there is no coverage of histograms, stem-leaf plots, box plots, dot plots, or other such techniques. Similarly, we focus on only the most basic summary measures of variable distributions and omit coverage of, say, the trimmed mean, the harmonic mean, the geometric mean, standard scores, etc. Instead, we have dedicated more space to the subjects that we deem most critical to an understanding of statistics as the discipline is practiced today: causality and causal inference, internal and external validity of statistical results, the sampling distribution of a statistic, the p value, common bivariate statistical procedures, multivariable modeling and the meaning of statistical control, and measures of the predictive efficacy of statistical models, to cite a few examples.

Along with this approach, we have avoided the extensive presentation of statistical formulas and sophisticated mathematics. Anyone with even a passing grasp of high-school algebra should have no trouble reading this primer. A few test-statistic formulas are shown to communicate the rationale underlying test statistics. Other than that, however, we simply name the tests that are used in different situations. Some algebraic formulas, however, are unavoidable. It is simply not possible to understand regression modeling in its different incarnations without showing regression equations. Similarly, growth-curve modeling and fixed-effects regression modeling are not understandable without their respective equations. Nevertheless, we have tried to explain, in the narrative, what these equations are conveying in an intuitive sense. And narrative is the operative word. This is not a traditional textbook; there are no exercises and no tables in the back. To the extent that such could be said about a statistics book, our intention was to make it a "good read."

A feature of the book that we think is especially useful is our extensive presentation of statistical applications from the recent medical literature. Over 30 different articles are explicated herein, taken from such journals as *Journal of the American Medical Association, Journal of Urology, British Journal of Urology International, American Journal of Epidemiology, Journal of Internal Medicine, Alcohol and Alcoholism,* and *BMC Neurology.* We deemed it important for readers to see how the various techniques covered in the primer are employed, displayed, and discussed in actual research. In the process we have attempted to "translate into English" some of the more recondite terminology used in the literature. Hopefully, this enterprise will facilitate the reader's understanding of statistical applications when he or she encounters them in the journals.

In the process of writing this primer, many people have been helpful to us. We wish, first, to acknowledge the kind guidance and cheerful flexibility of Marc Strauss, our editor at Springer. We also wish to thank Bowling Green State University, in particular the Center for Family and Demographic Research, as well as the University of Toledo Medical Center, for providing the computer and library support that made this work possible. Also deserving of thanks are Annette Mahoney and Kenneth I. Pargament in the Psychology Department at Bowling Green State University for collecting the NAPPS data that are drawn on extensively in Chap. 9. And last, but certainly not least, we wish to gratefully acknowledge our wives, Gabrielle and Linda, for the loving support and encouragement they provided during the writing of this work. And now, let us begin...

Bowling Green, OH, USA   Alfred DeMaris
Toledo, OH, USA   Steven H. Selman

Contents

Chapter 1
Statistics and Causality

What Is Statistics?

Question: What's the difference between accountants and statisticians?
Answer: Well, they both work with numbers, but statisticians just don't have the personality to be accountants.

Such is the stereotype of statisticians and statistics. Dull, plodding, and concerned with the tedious bean-counting enterprise of compiling numbers and tables and graphs on topics nobody much cares about. Nothing could be further from the truth. Well, okay, statisticians *are* dull; but statistics is one of the most exciting disciplines of all. Like astronomy, it's an investigation of the unknown—and, possibly, *unknowable*—world that's largely invisible to the naked eye. But this world is the one right under our noses: in terms of the subject of this book, it consists of human beings and their health. In this first chapter, we will consider what statistics is and why it is essential to the medical enterprise, and to science in general. Here, we define the science of statistics and relate it to real-world medical problems. Medical research is typically concerned with cause-and-effect relationships. The causes of disease or of health problems are important, as are the causal effects of treatments on medical outcomes. Therefore, we also discuss in this chapter the notion of a causal effect, and we ponder the conditions necessary for inferring causality in research.

What Statistics Is

Statistics is the science of converting data into evidence. *Data* constitute the raw material of statistics. They consist of numbers, letters, or special characters representing measurements of properties made on a collection of cases. Cases are the units of analysis in our study. Cases are usually people, but they could be days of

A. DeMaris and S.H. Selman, *Converting Data into Evidence: A Statistics Primer for the Medical Practitioner*, DOI 10.1007/978-1-4614-7792-1_1,

the week, organizations, nations or, in meta-analyses, other published studies. *Evidence* refers to information pertinent to judging the truth or falsehood of an assertion. The heart of statistics is called *inferential* statistics. It's concerned with making inferences about some population of cases. To do that, it uses a sample drawn from that population of cases and studies *it* rather than the entire population. On the basis of findings from the sample, we estimate some characteristic of a population or we judge the plausibility of statements made about the population. Let's take an example.

An Example

A frequent interest in medical research is HIV transmission and the course of the disease for those who are so infected (see, for example, Bendavid et al. 2012; Paton et al. 2012). Suppose a team of medical researchers is interested in the association between recreational intravenous drug use (IVDU) and contracting HIV in the USA. They believe that needle sharing is the prime means of transmission of this disease among the IVDU population. So they want to estimate the proportion of that population who is involved in needle sharing, for one thing. Then they want to test the hypothesis that needle sharing is a risk factor for becoming HIV positive (HIV+). But if they find that needle sharing is, in fact, associated with an elevated risk for HIV+, they want to ensure that it is the practice of sharing needles that is the "driver" of this association. That is, they need to rule out the possibility that it is some other risky behavior associated with sharing needles that is actually causing the association. Examples of other risky behaviors possibly associated with both IVDU and needle sharing are having unprotected sex, having sex with multiple partners, poor hygiene practices, and so forth.

This research problem presents several dilemmas. First, the population of interest is *all recreational IV drug users in the USA*. Now, what do you think the chances are of finding that population, let alone studying it? That's right—zip. Most users would not admit to having a drug habit, so we're unlikely to get very far surveying the USA population and asking people to self-identify as recreational IV drug users. So our let's say our team manages to recruit a sample of drug users, perhaps through a newspaper or magazine advertisement offering financial remuneration for taking part in a study. They find that 50 % of the sample of IV drug users share needles with other users. At this point the researchers would like to use this figure as their estimate of the proportion of all IV drug users in the USA who share needles. How should they proceed? Let's recognize, first, that the population proportion in question is a summary measure that statisticians refer to as a *parameter*. A parameter is just a summary statistic measuring some aspect of a population. Second, the parameter is unknown, and, in fact, *unknowable*. It's not possible to measure it directly, even though it exists "out there," somewhere. The best the team can do is to estimate it and then figure out how that estimate relates to the actual parameter value. We will spend much of this first part of the book on how this is accomplished.

Next, in order to test the primary hypothesis about needle sharing being a cause of HIV+status, there has to be a comparison group of non-IV drug users. These individuals are much easier to find, since most people don't engage in IVDU. Let's say the team also recruits a control sample of such individuals, matched with the IVDU group on gender, age, race, and education. They then need to measure all the relevant variables. This includes the "mechanisms," aside from needle sharing, that they believe might be responsible for the IVDU-HIV+association, i.e., having unprotected sex, having sex with multiple partners, quality of personal hygiene, and so forth. In order to fully evaluate the hypothesis, they will conduct a *multivariable analysis* (or *multivariate analysis*—these terms are used interchangeably). HIV+status will be the primary *study endpoint* (or *response variable*), and needle sharing and the other risky behaviors will be the *explanatory variables* (or *regressors, predictors,* or *covariates*). The multivariable analysis will allow them to examine whether needle sharing is responsible for the (presumed) higher HIV+rate among the IVDU vs. the non-IVDU group. It will also let them assess whether it is needle sharing, per se, rather than one of the other risky behaviors that is the driving factor. We will discuss multivariable statistical techniques in a later section of the book.

However, there are other complications to be dealt with. Suppose that some of the subjects of the study fail to provide answers to some of the questions? This creates the problem of *missing data.* We can simply discard these subjects from the study, but then we (a) lose all of the other information that they did provide and (b) introduce selection bias into the study because those who don't answer items are usually not just a random subset of the subjects. This means that those left in the sample are a select group—perhaps a more compliant type of individuals—and the results then will only apply to people of that type. One solution is that the researchers can *impute* the missing data and then still include the cases. Imputation is the practice of filling in the missing data with a value representing our best guess about what the missing value would be were it measured. The state of the art in imputation techniques is a procedure called *multiple imputation.* Multiple imputation will be covered later in the book in the chapter on advanced techniques.

The last major issue is that it's always possible that some characteristic that the researchers have not measured might be producing the association between needle sharing and HIV+status. That is, it's not really needle sharing that elevates HIV+risk. It's some unmeasured characteristic of individuals that also happens to be associated with needle sharing. An unmeasured characteristic that may be influencing one's results is often referred to as *unmeasured heterogeneity.* The term refers to the fact that the characteristic exhibits heterogeneity—i.e., variance—across individuals that is related to the variation in the study endpoint. The fact that it is unmeasured means that there is no easy way to control for it in our analyses. We will discuss this problem in greater detail later in this chapter. And we will see one possible statistical solution to this problem, called *fixed-effects regression modeling,* when we get to the advanced techniques chapter. In sum, statistics allows us to address research problems of the foregoing nature and provide answers to these kinds of complex questions that are posed routinely in research.

Populations and Samples

The population in any study is the *total collection of cases we want to make assertions about*. A "case" is the smallest element constituting a single "replication" of a treatment. Suppose, for example, that you are interested in the effect of diet on prostate-specific antigen (PSA). You suspect that a diet heavy in red meat contains carcinogens that raise the risk for prostate cancer. So you anticipate that a red-meat-rich diet will be associated with higher PSA levels. Suppose you have a sample of six men from each of two groups: a control group eating a balanced diet and a treatment group eating a diet overloaded with red meat. In this case, individual men are the cases, since each man eating a particular diet represents a replication of the "treatment." By "treatment," in this case, we mean diet, of which there are two treatment levels: balanced and red-meat rich. Who is the population here? The population we'd ideally like to be talking about is the entire population of adult males in the USA. So our 12 men constitute a sample from it.

Probability vs. Nonprobability Samples

Statisticians distinguish two major classes of samples: probability and nonprobability. A *probability sample* is one for which one can specify the probability that any member of the population will be selected into it. *Nonprobability samples* do not have this property. The best-known probability sample is a simple random sample or SRS. An SRS is one in which every member of the population has the same chance of being selected into the sample. For example, if the population consists of 50,000 units and we're drawing an SRS of 50 units from it, each population member has a 50/50,000=0.001 chance of being selected. Probability samples provide results that can be generalized to the population. Nonprobability samples don't. In our diet study example, if the 12 men were randomly sampled from the population of interest, the results could be generalized to that population. Most likely, though, the 12 men were recruited via advertisement or by virtue of being part of a patient population. If the 12 men weren't sampled randomly "from" a known population, then what kind of population might they represent?

Sampling "to" a Population

Many samples in science are of the nonprobability type. What can we say about the "population" of interest, then? Some statisticians will tell you: nothing. But that implies that your sample is so unique, there's no one else who behaves or responds the same way to a treatment. That's not very realistic. Rather, what we can do with nonprobability sample results is use the characteristics of sample participants to suggest a hypothetical population the results might be generalizable to. Much of the time in studies of this nature, the sample consists of volunteers responding to a newspaper ad announcing a clinical trial. In research involving the human body, one could, of course, argue that people are sufficiently similar biologically that the 12 men in the example above are representative of men in general. But statistically, at least, generalizing to a population requires sampling randomly from it. Another way to define the population, however, is to reason in the opposite direction. That is, whatever the manner in which the 12 men were recruited for this study, suppose we repeat that recruitment strategy and collect 12 men a second time. And suppose we repeat it, again, and collect a third group of 12 men. And then suppose we go on and on like this, collecting sample after sample of 12 men by repeating the recruitment strategy over and over, ad infinitum. Eventually, the entire collection of men accumulating from all of these samples could be considered the "population." And our original sample of 12 men can then be thought of as a random sample from *this* population. This has been termed "sampling *to* a population," as opposed to sampling *from* a population (DeMaris 2004), and is one way of defining a conceptual population that one's inferences might apply to.

Statistics and Causal Inference

The scientific enterprise is typically concerned with cause and effect. What causes elevated PSA levels, for example? Or, what causes prostate cancer? Or, what causes prostate cancer to develop sooner rather than later? Statistics can aid in making causal inferences. To understand its utility in this arena, however, we first have to define what we mean by "cause," or, more properly, a "causal effect." The reigning definition in contemporary science is due to two statisticians, Jerzy Neyman and Donald Rubin (West and Thoemmes 2010). The Neyman–Rubin causal paradigm is simple, mathematically elegant, and intuitive. We normally think of a cause as something that changes life's "trajectory" from what would have transpired were the cause not operating. The Neyman–Rubin paradigm simply puts this in mathematical terms.

A Mathematical Definition of "Causal Effect"

Employing, again, the diet-PSA example, suppose a man follows a balanced diet for some period of time. His PSA level measured after that period would be denoted Yc. And then suppose he were instead to follow a meat-heavy diet for the same period. Denote his PSA level after that as Yt. Notice that this scenario is *contrary to fact*. He can't follow both diets over the same period; he's either on one or the other. But suspend disbelief for a moment and suppose that's what he does. The causal effect of the steak diet on PSA is defined as: Yt−Yc. It is the boost in PSA attributable to the steak diet. So if his PSA is 2.6 on the balanced diet vs. 4.3 on the steak diet, the causal effect of diet is $4.3 - 2.6 = 1.7$, or the steak diet results in a boost in PSA level by 1.7.

If we were to apply this regimen to every man in the population and then average all of the $(Yt - Yc)$ differences, we would have the *Average Causal Effect*, or ACE, of the steak diet on PSA. The ACE is often the *parameter* of interest in research. If the outcome of interest is a qualitative one, then the true causal effect is defined with a slightly different measure. So if the man in question has a 30 % chance of developing prostate cancer on the balanced diet, but a 60 % chance on the steak diet, the causal effect of a steak diet on the risk of cancer is $0.60/0.30 = 2$. Or, a steak diet doubles the risk of cancer for this particular man. The number 2 is called the *relative risk* for cancer due to a steak, vs. a balanced, diet.

How Do We Estimate the ACE?

Because the ACE is contrary-to-fact, and therefore not measurable, how can we estimate it? It turns out that the ACE can be estimated in an unbiased fashion as the mean difference in PSA levels between men on a balanced vs. a meat diet in a study if a particular condition is met. The condition is referred to as the *ignorability* condition: the treatment assignment mechanism is ignorable if the potential outcomes (e.g., PSA levels) are independent of the treatment assignment "mechanism." What this means in practice, using our example, is that there is no a priori tendency for those in the steak-diet condition to have higher or lower PSA levels than men in the other condition *before the treatments are even applied*. The only way to ensure this is to *randomly assign* the men to the two diet conditions, and this is the hallmark of the clinical trial, or, for that matter, any experimental study. Random assignment to treatment groups ensures that, *on average*, treatment and control groups are exactly the same on all characteristics at the beginning of a study. In this manner, we are assured that the treatment effect is a true causal effect and is not an artifact of a latent *self-selection factor*. It is random assignment to treatment levels that provides researchers with the best vehicle for inferring causality.

Example of Latent Self-Selection

As an example of latent self-selection confounding causal inference in a study, regard Fig. 1.1, below. It shows one possible scenario that could occur in the absence of random assignment, such as if we simply study groups of men who have chosen each type of diet themselves.

The negative numbers represent inverse relationships. The "−0.75" on the curved arrow connecting health awareness with meat diet is a *correlation coefficient*. It means those with greater health awareness are less likely to be on a meat diet. They

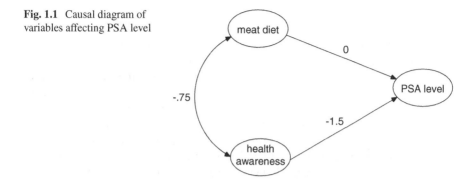

Fig. 1.1 Causal diagram of variables affecting PSA level

are probably men who lead healthy lifestyles that include moderate alcohol intake, nonsmoking, plenty of exercise, regular medical checkups, etc. The "−1.5" from health awareness to PSA levels is a *causal effect*. It means that health awareness leads to lower PSA levels. Simply looking at the difference in average PSA between the two groups of men while ignoring health awareness confounds the true relationship of diet to PSA. There might be no association of diet with PSA (shown by the "0" on that path in the diagram). But if health awareness is not "controlled" in the study, then the indirect link from meat diet to PSA level through health awareness will manifest itself as a positive "effect" of a meat diet on PSA level. This happens because ignoring health awareness is equivalent to multiplying together the two negative numbers: $(-0.75) \times (-1.5) = 1.125$, and then adding the result to the path from meat diet to PSA level. This makes it appear that meat diet has a positive effect on PSA level: the "1.125" would appear to be the average PSA level difference between the men in the two groups. The take-home message here is simple: only random assignment to treatment conditions lets us confidently rule out latent selection factors as accounting for treatment effects in a study. In epidemiological and other observational—as opposed to experimental—studies, latent selection factors are an ever-present threat. They are typically countered by measuring any such selection factors ahead of time, and then statistically controlling for them when estimating causal effects. Under the right conditions, we can even eliminate *unmeasured* factors, as we shall see in the advanced techniques chapter. And we shall have more to say about statistical control, in general, later in this primer.

Internal vs. External Validity: A Conundrum

At this point, we have discussed the nature of causal effects, the advantages of random assignment to treatment conditions, and latent selection factors in nonexperimental studies. It is worth noting, as a final issue, that both experimental and nonexperimental studies have particular advantages and drawbacks. And both are regularly used in medical research. Statisticians speak of a study having internal vs. external validity. *Internal validity* obtains to the extent that the treatment-group differences observed on a study endpoint strictly represent the causal effect of the treatment on the response variable (Singleton and Straits 2010). *External validity* obtains to the extent that the study's results can be generalized to a larger, known population. As we have noted, experimental studies, in which cases are randomly assigned to treatment groups, are ideal for estimating causal effects. The gold standard in this genre is the double-blind, placebo-controlled, clinical trial. Studies of this nature have a clear advantage in internal validity over nonexperimental studies. However, experimental studies may be deficient in external validity. For one thing, it may not be clear what population the study results are generalizable to. It is very rare—in fact, unheard of—for researchers to take a random sample of a patient population and then randomly assign sample members to treatment conditions. Patients are usually a "captive audience"; they are at hand by virtue of seeking treatment from a given clinic or hospital. Or they are recruited through advertisements for a clinical trial. As they don't typically represent a probability sample from a known population, it is not immediately clear what larger population they might represent. We can invoke the aforementioned notion of "sampling to a population" to justify a kind of generalizability. But the larger population the results might apply to is only hypothetical. A second factor that detracts from external validity is that, in actual clinical practice, patients are not randomly assigned to treatments. They elect to undergo certain treatments in consultation with their physician. Therefore, there is always an element of self-selection operating in the determination of which patients end up getting which treatments. This may lead to a different treatment outcome than if patients were randomly assigned to their treatments (Marcus et al. 2012). Thus, the pure causal effect observed in a clinical trial may not correspond perfectly to the real-world patient setting.

Nonexperimental studies often have an advantage in external validity. Many nonexperimental studies are based on probability sampling from a known population. Moreover, many follow patients after they have undergone treatments of their own choosing—on physician advice, of course. The disadvantage, as noted previously, is that nonexperimental study results can always be confounded by unmeasured heterogeneity. It is never possible to control for all possible patient characteristics that might affect the study results. Hence, nonexperimental studies often suffer from questions regarding their internal validity. We shall have much more to say about nonexperimental data analysis in subsequent chapters. In the meantime, the next chapter introduces techniques for summarizing the main features of a set of data. Understanding what your data "look like" is a first step in the research process.

Chapter 2
Summarizing Data

Descriptive Statistical Techniques

In this chapter we discuss how to use *descriptive statistical techniques,* or techniques employed for data description, for summarizing the *sample distribution* of a variable. Interest will primarily revolve around two tasks. The first is finding the *center* of the distribution, which tells us what the typical or average score in the distribution is. The most commonly employed measure of center is the arithmetic average, or *mean*, of the distribution. The second task is assessing the *dispersion*, or degree of spread of the values, in the distribution. This indicates how much variability there is in the values of the variable of interest. Additionally, we will learn about *percentiles* and another important measure of center: the *median*. Finally, we expand the discussion to considering the characteristics of the *population distribution* on a variable. But first we must distinguish between *quantitative* vs. *qualitative* variables.

Quantitative vs. Qualitative Data

Data come in different forms. One basic distinction is whether the data are *quantitative* or *qualitative*. Quantitative data are represented by numbers that indicate the exact amount of the characteristic present. Alternatively, they may simply indicate a "rank order" of units according to the amount of the characteristic present. By "rank order" is meant a ranking from lowest to highest on the characteristic of interest. So weight in pounds is a quantitative variable indicating the exact weight of an individual. Degree of pain experienced, on a 0–10 scale, is also quantitative. But the numbers don't represent exactly how much pain is present. Rather they represent a rank order on pain, so that someone who circles 8 is presumed to be in more pain than if they circled 7, and so forth. In statistics, we will typically treat quantitative

A. DeMaris and S.H. Selman, *Converting Data into Evidence: A Statistics Primer for the Medical Practitioner*, DOI 10.1007/978-1-4614-7792-1_2,
© Springer Science+Business Media New York 2013

Control	Steak	Vegetarian
4.6	2.0	1.7
2.3	4.9	2.1
2.7	3.1	1.6
3.0	2.6	4.2
6.0	7.0	3.0
4.0	7.5	4.7

Table 2.1 PSA levels for men in the diet-PSA study

data the same, regardless of their "exactness," provided there are enough different levels of the variable to work with. Five levels are usually enough if the sample is not too small.

Qualitative data, in statistical parlance, refers to data whose values differ only qualitatively. That is, the different values of a qualitative variable represent differences in type only, and bear no quantitative relation to each other. Examples are gender, race, region of residence, country of origin, political party preference, blood type, eye color, etc. Normally, we use numbers to represent qualitative data, too. But in their case, the numbers are just labels and convey no quantitative meaning. So, for example, gender can be represented using 1 for males and 2 for females. But it is a qualitative variable; the numbers do not indicate either the "amount of gender" present or "rank order" on gender. The numbers are just labels; they could just as well be letters or smiley faces. (Numbers are most convenient, however, for computer manipulation.) Qualitative data call for different statistical techniques, compared to quantitative data, as we will see in this primer.

Describing Data

Table 2.1 presents PSA levels for three groups of men who were randomly assigned to follow either a control diet (a diet balanced in meat, vegetables, fruits, etc.), a steak diet, or a vegetarian diet for 6 months. At the end of that period, their PSA was measured.

Measuring Center and Spread of a Variable's Distribution

The Mean

The *distribution* of a variable is an enumeration or depiction of all of its values. The distribution of PSA in each group is readily apparent in the table. Two important features of distributions are the *central tendency* and *dispersion* of the variable. Central tendency describes where the "center" of the data is. Intuitively, it is a measure of what the typical value in the distribution is, and is most often captured with the *mean* or arithmetic average. Most of us are already familiar with the mean. It's just the sum of the values of a variable divided by the total number of values. So the mean PSA for the steak-diet group is:

$$\text{Mean(PSA)} = \frac{(2.0 + 4.9 + 3.1 + 2.6 + 7.0 + 7.5)}{6} = 4.52.$$

The mean is interpreted thus: average PSA in the steak-diet group is 4.52.

Percentiles and the Median

Another measure of central tendency that is often used is the *median*. To define this measure we first define percentiles: the pth percentile is that value in the distribution such that p percent of the values are that value or lower than that value in the distribution, and $1-p$ percent are greater than that value. To describe a distribution's percentiles, we have to order the values from smallest to largest. For the steak-diet group, the ordered PSA values are 2.0, 2.6, 3.1, 4.9, 7.0, 7.5. There are six unique values here, and each one therefore constitutes 1/6 or 16.7 % of the distribution. So the 16.7th percentile of the distribution is 2.0. That is, 16.7 % of the PSA values are ≤ 2.0. The 33.4th percentile is 2.6, since 33.4 % of the PSA values are ≤ 2.6 and so forth. The median is the 50th percentile of the distribution. That is, it's the value that is in the exact middle of the distribution. With an even number of values, as in this case, the median is taken to be the average of the two middle values. So the median of the PSA values is $(3.1+4.9)/2=4$. It is easy to see that 50 % of the PSA values are ≤ 4 and 50 % of the PSA values are >4. Two other commonly referenced percentiles are the *first quartile*, which is the score such that 25 % of scores are less than or equal to it, and the *third quartile*, which is the score such that 75 % of the scores are less than or equal to it. The median is often used to describe a distribution's center when the distribution is skewed or lopsided. For example, the average income for US households is typically described using the median rather than the mean. Why? Well, the majority of people have modest incomes. A relatively small proportion have really large incomes, say, several million dollars per year. If we use the mean income to describe the typical household, it will be unrealistically large. The problem is that the mean is usually "pulled" in the direction of the extreme cases, compared to the median. Instead, using the median will give us an income value that is closer to what most households earn.

Dispersion

The other important feature is *dispersion* or the degree to which the data are spread out. Dispersion, or variability, is an extremely important property of data. We can't find causes for things that don't vary. For example, we can't explain why everyone eventually dies. There's no variability, because…well, everybody dies. But we can study what affects the timing of death, because there's variability in that. And we can try to understand why people die from this or that condition, because that also shows variation.

One way to measure dispersion is via the variable's *range*, which is simply the maximum value minus the minimum value. For the steak-diet condition, the range of PSA is $7.5 - 2 = 5.5$. The range is not all that useful, however. Much more useful would be a measure that tells how well the mean represents the values in the dataset. That is, are most values similar to the mean, or are they very spread out on either side of it? The measure statisticians use is approximately the average distance of the units from the mean. We say "approximately" because it's not literally the average distance. Why not? Well, suppose we were to calculate the average distance from the mean for the PSA values of the steak-diet group. We need to subtract the mean from each value and then average the result. We get the following *deviations* of each value from the mean:

$2 - 4.52 = -2.52$
$4.9 - 4.52 = 0.38$
$3.1 - 4.52 = -1.42$
$2.6 - 4.52 = -1.92$
$7.0 - 4.52 = 2.48$
$7.5 - 4.52 = 2.98$

Now if we sum these values so that we can get the average, we have:

$$-2.52 + 0.38 + (-1.42) + (-1.92) + 2.48 + 2.98 = -0.02.$$

Notice that the positives and negatives tend to cancel out, so the sum is approximately zero. In fact, it's exactly zero if no rounding is used in the mean (the mean is actually 4.516666…). *And this will always be the case.* Hence, to eliminate the signs on these deviations from the mean, we square each deviation and then add up the squared deviations:

$$\text{Sum of squared deviations} = (-2.52)^2 + (0.38)^2 + (-1.42)^2 + (-1.92)^2$$
$$+ (2.48)^2 + (2.98)^2$$
$$= 27.228.$$

We then divide by 5 to get, roughly, the "average" squared deviation. *Dividing by 5 instead of 6 gives us an unbiased estimate of the corresponding "population" parameter.* Unbiasedness is explained below. The result is called the *sample variance*, and is denoted by "s^2":

$$s^2 = \frac{27.228}{5} = 5.45.$$

Table 2.2 Distribution of physician stewardship for 2,746 respondents in the 2002 GSS

RELYDOC	R RELIES ON DOCTOR'S KNOWLEDGE

Description of the Variable

854. I will read you some statements of beliefs people have.
Please look at the card and decide which answer best applies to
you. c. I prefer to rely on my doctor's knowledge and not try to
find out about my condition on my own.

Percent	N	Value	Label
26.0	715	1	Strongly disagree
15.0	413	2	Moderately disagree
14.5	399	3	Slightly disagree
12.6	345	4	Slightly agree
16.5	453	5	Moderately agree
15.3	421	6	Strongly agree
	52,322	0	IAP
	14	8	DONT KNOW
	5	9	NO ANSWER
100.0	55,087		Total

Finally, we take the square root of the variance to get the measure of dispersion we're after. It's called the *standard deviation* and is denoted "s":

$$s = \sqrt{5.45} = 2.33.$$

The standard deviation is interpreted as the *average distance from the mean in the set of values*. So the average man in the steak-diet group is 2.33 PSA units away from the mean of 4.52. Knowing the minimum and maximum value, the mean, and the standard deviation for a set of values usually gives us a pretty good picture of its distribution.

Data from the General Social Survey

As another example of sample data we consider the 2002 General Social Survey (GSS). The GSS is a national probability sample of the USA noninstitutionalized adult population that has been conducted approximately every other year since 1972. The sample size each time has been around 2,000 respondents. To date there is a total of around 55,000 respondents who have been surveyed. In 2002 the sample size was 2,765 respondents. That year, the GSS asked a few questions about people's attitudes toward physicians (Table 2.2). Here is one of the questions (it's the third question in a series; that's why it's preceded by "c."):

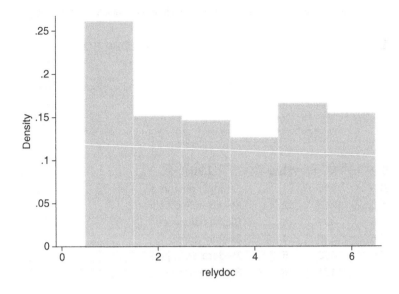

Fig. 2.1 Bar graph of physician stewardship (Relydoc) for respondents in the 2002 GSS

Notice that this is a quantitative variable in which the values represent rank order on the dimension of interest, which we shall call "physician stewardship." The higher the value, the more the respondent is willing to let the doctor exercise stewardship over his or her medical condition. Three of the codes are not counted toward the percent breakdown. "IAP" means "inapplicable." As this question was only asked in the 2002 survey, GSS respondents from other years are given this code. A few respondents in 2002, however either said they "don't know" (code 8) or they refused to answer the question (code 9). The "N" column shows how many respondents gave each response. The total number of valid responses (for which a percent is given) is 2,746 (not shown). The mean of this variable is 3.24 (not shown), which falls about a quarter of the way between "slightly disagree" and "slightly agree." That is, on average, respondents had a slight preference for finding out about their condition on their own. The standard deviation is 1.82 (also not shown). The mean and standard deviation would be computed in the manner shown above, but involving 2,746 individual cases. Fortunately, we have let the computer do that work for us.

Although the standard deviation is the preferred measure of spread, it's not always obvious how much spread is indicated by its value. One way to decipher that is to realize that the most the standard deviation can be is one-half of the range. In this case, that would be 2.5. So the standard deviation of 1.82 is 1.82/2.5 = 0.73 or 73 % of its maximum value. This suggests quite a bit of spread, as is evident from Fig. 2.1. This figure shows a bar graph of the variable's distribution (the proportion of the sample having a particular value is shown by the "Density" on the vertical axis). The length of each bar represents the proportion of respondents giving each response. The variable's name, for software purposes, is "relydoc."

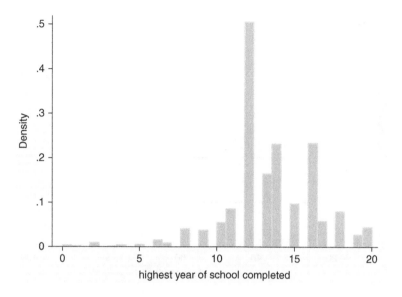

Fig. 2.2 Bar graph of education for respondents in the 2002 GSS

Next, Fig. 2.2 shows a bar graph for respondent education, in number of years of schooling completed, for the GSS respondents.

The *n* (number of valid respondents) for this variable is 2,753 (not shown). As is evident, the range is 0–20. The mean is 13.36 (not shown) and the standard deviation is 2.97 (not shown). The tallest bar in about the middle of the graph here is for 12 years of schooling, representing a high-school education. The mean of 13.36 suggests that, on average, respondents have had about a year and a third of college. This distribution is notably *skewed to the left*. That is, the bulk of the data falls between education levels of 10–20, but a few "outliers" have as few years of schooling as 0–5.

Figure 2.3 presents a bar graph of the distribution of age for respondents in the 2002 GSS.

Here, the *n* is 2,751 (not shown); the mean is 46.28 (not shown), and the standard deviation is 17.37 (not shown). The ages range from 18 to 89. In contrast to education, the distribution of age is somewhat *skewed to the right*.

Describing the Population Distribution

What we are really interested in is not the sample, but the population. The sample is just a vehicle for making inferences about the population. A quantitative variable's distribution in the population is of utmost importance. Why? Well, for one thing, it determines how likely one is to observe particular values of the variable in a sample.

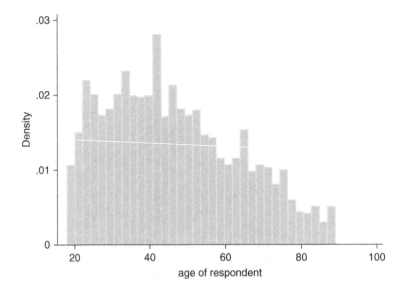

Fig. 2.3 Bar graph of age for respondents in the 2002 GSS

The population distribution for a variable, "X," is simply a depiction of all of the different values X can take in the population, along with their proportionate representation in the distribution. It is just the population analog of the variable's distribution in the sample. It would be impossible to show all the individual values of X in the population, because populations are generally very large. For example, the US population is well over 300 million people. Therefore, population distributions for quantitative variables are depicted as smooth curves over a horizontal line representing the range of the variable's values. The form of the age distribution immediately above already suggests this kind of representation.

Figure 2.4 depicts a distribution for some variable "X" in a population. As an example, the population could be all adult men in the USA, and the variable X could be PSA level.

In this figure, the horizontal axis shows the values of X, and the vertical axis shows the probability associated with those values. The distribution is again right-skewed. This means that most of the X values are in the left half of the figure, say, to the left of about 7 on the horizontal axis. But there is an elongated "tail" of the distribution on the right with a few extreme values in it. That is, the distribution is "skewed" to the right.

The height of the curve corresponds to the proportion of units that have the particular value of X directly under it. So the proportion that have a value of 5, say, is substantially greater than those having a value of 10. Because the total area under the curve is equal to 1.0, the proportion of the area corresponding to a range of X values, such as the area between "a" and "b" in the figure, is equal to the probability of observing those values when you sample one unit from the population. The

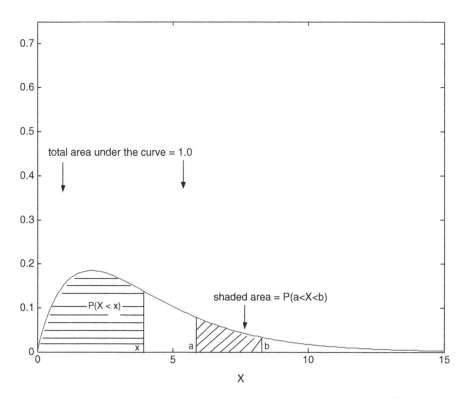

Fig. 2.4 Population distribution for a variable, X. Reprinted with permission from John Wiley & Sons, Publishers, from DeMaris (2004)

probability of observing a value between a and b, denoted "$P(a<x<b)$," is shown as the shaded area to the right. The probability of observing a value less than "x" on the horizontal line, denoted "$P(X<x)$," is the shaded area on the left, and so on.

The Normal and t Distributions

Frequently in biologic and medical science, data describing the way a variable is distributed in the population assume a bell-shaped configuration. This configuration, or distribution, is called the *normal distribution*. The normal distribution is arguably the most important distribution in statistics. The reason is not so much because real-world data follow this pattern, but because it characterizes the sampling distribution of many a statistical measure. We shall have much more to say about sampling distributions below. In the meantime, Fig. 2.5 depicts the normal distribution, along with its close relative, the *t distribution*.

These distributions are symmetric. This means that exactly 50 % of the distribution is on either side of the mean, which for both of these distributions is zero in this

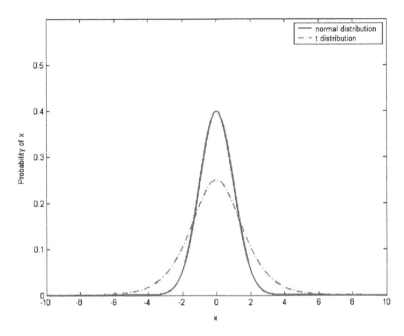

Fig. 2.5 The normal and *t* distributions

instance. It also means that the area to the right of any value, say 4, is exactly equal to the area to the left of the negative of that value, i.e. –4, and so on. The standard deviation of the normal distribution shown here is 1. The standard deviation of the *t* distribution is greater; it's 1.8. And it is clear in the figure that the *t* distribution is somewhat more spread out than the normal. The *t* distribution has an associated *degrees of freedom* or df (a technical concept that we won't go into here; just note that every *t* distribution requires a df to fully characterize it). This particular *t* distribution has 7 df. It turns out that when the df gets large enough, the *t* distribution becomes indistinguishable from the normal distribution. You may have heard of the "*t* test" in statistics. The *t* test, which is discussed in Chap. 4, is a test of whether two groups have the same mean on a study endpoint. That test is so named because it relies on the *t* distribution. In fact, several tests in statistics rely on this useful distribution.

A normal distribution is distinguished by the proportions of its values that are within certain distances from the mean. For example, approximately 68 % of values are within one standard deviation from the mean, approximately 95 % are within two standard deviations, and almost all of the values are within three standard deviations. Moreover, we can determine the probability of a value being more than some distance from the mean. For example, only 2.5 % of the values are more than 1.96 standard deviations above the mean. Similarly, only 2.5 % of the values are more than 1.96 standard deviations below the mean. And this means that *exactly 95 % of all values are within 1.96 standard deviations on either side of the mean* (1.96 is approximately 2 standard deviations). This type of information will be very useful when we discuss confidence intervals (below).

The other reason why population distributions are important is that their parameters are often the subject of inference. For example, we often want to know what the mean of the distribution is. In general, the population mean is symbolized by μ, and is calculated the same way as the sample mean, except using the entire population. More to the point, we may want to know if population means for different groups are different in value. Remember that in the diet-PSA study we anticipate that mean PSA for the population of men exposed to a steak diet is higher than mean PSA for the population of men exposed to a balanced diet. In the next chapter, we will consider how to test this hypothesis. In the meantime, let's see how descriptive statistics are used to describe the characteristics of samples in actual medical studies.

Applications: Descriptive Statistics in Action

Medical studies typically present a table showing the demographic and medical characteristics of the subjects in their sample. Descriptive statistics are presented to illuminate the medical/personal profile of the typical sample member. At times figures are presented to illustrate particular patterns exhibited by the study's findings. In what follows, we offer a sampling of descriptive results from different studies.

Tarenflurbil Study

A study by Green et al. (2009) that appeared in *The Journal of the American Medical Association* was concerned with the degree of cognitive decline in patients with mild Alzheimer disease. In this clinical trial, the researchers tested the ability of tarenflurbil, a selective $A\beta_{42}$-lowering agent, to slow the rate of decline in patients with mild Alzheimer disease. Across 133 participating trial sites, patients were randomly assigned either to tarenflurbil or placebo treatment groups for an 18-month period. Characteristics of the study subjects were described in Table 1 of the article. For example, mean age of subjects in the placebo and tarenflurbil groups was 74.7 and 74.6, respectively. Standard deviations of age in each group were 8.4 and 8.5, respectively, and age ranges were 53–100 in each group. Not surprisingly, randomization has created groups with equivalent age distributions. The proportion of females, on the other hand, was slightly higher in the placebo group (52.5 %) compared to the tarenflurbil group (49.4 %). This difference however was not "statistically significant," a term to be discussed in the next chapter. In fact, none of the patient characteristics, including measures of pre-randomization cognitive functioning, were meaningfully different between the two groups. Thus, the randomization for this study was successfully executed.

Hydroxychloroquine Study

Sometimes researchers, in describing the characteristics of the sample, will employ the median and the *interquartile range* (IQR) for describing center and spread of a variable's distribution, rather than the mean and standard deviation. The IQR is simply the interval from the first to the third quartile. For example, Paton et al. (2012) studied whether the agent hydroxychloroquine might be good for decreasing immune activation and inflammation and thereby slow the progression of early HIV disease. Their study was a randomized clinical trial comparing hydroxychloroquine 400 mg vs placebo once daily for 48 weeks. The primary endpoint was the change from baseline to week 48 in activation of CD8 cells. In their table of baseline characteristics (Table 1), they report the median (IQR) for time since HIV diagnosis as 3.0 (1.7–5.6) years for the hydroxycholoroquine group and 2.5 (1.7–3.5) years for the placebo group. The median and IQR would be preferred measures of center and spread, respectively, when variable distributions were particularly skewed. In this study, it was not clear that such was the case, but apparently median and IQR were used anyway.

RALP Study

Yu et al. (2012) undertook a study of the utilization rates at different hospitals of robot-assisted laparoscopic radical prostatectomy (RALP), along with associated patterns of care and patient outcomes due to the procedure. They used the nationwide inpatient sample (NIS), which is a 20 % stratified probability sample of hospital stays consisting of about eight million acute hospital stays annually from more than 1,000 hospitals in 42 states. During the last quarter of 2008 there were 2,093,300 subjects in NIS. A total of 2,348 RALPs are included in the NIS (Yu et al. 2012). RALP surgical volumes characterizing different hospitals are grouped into categories ranging from 1–5 surgeries to a maximum of 166–170 surgeries. Figure 2.6 shows a distribution of the percent of hospitals falling into each RALP surgical-volume category.

   The distribution depicted in Fig. 2.6 is very clearly right-skewed. Most hospitals have RALP surgical volumes between 1–5 and 31–35. A few, however, have RALP surgical volumes as high as 96–100 and 166–70. For example, the *modal* (i.e., the most common) surgical volume is 11–15 RALPs. 20.9 % of hospitals have this level of surgical volume. At the other extreme, only 0.9 % of hospitals perform as many as 166–170 RALPs.

Brachytherapy Study

Emara et al. (2011) employed graphic techniques to describe the effect of treatment on the primary study endpoint in their study. Their research evaluated the urinary and bowel symptoms, quality of life, and sexual function of men followed for 5–10 years after treatment with low-dose rate brachytherapy for prostate cancer at their

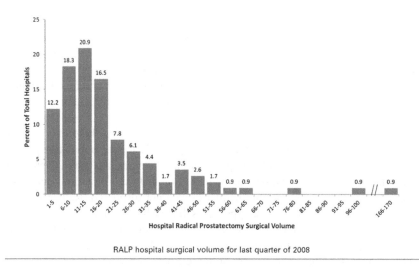

RALP hospital surgical volume for last quarter of 2008

Fig. 2.6 Percent distribution of hospitals falling into each RALP surgical-volume category. Reprinted with permission of Elsevier Publishers from Yu et al. (2012)

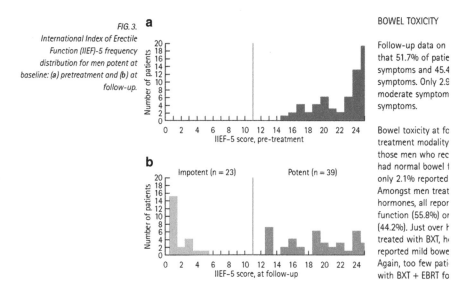

Fig. 2.7 Distribution of (IIEF)-5 scores before vs. after brachytherapy for prostate cancer. Reprinted with permission from John Wiley & Sons, Publishers, from Emara et al. (2011)

cancer center. Sexual function was assessed with the International Index of Erectile Function (IIEF)-5 scale. This measure has scores ranging from 1 to 25, with higher scores signifying better erectile function. Men with scores ≥11 were considered "potent." Figure 2.7 shows the distribution of (IIEF)-5 scores for the men prior to their cancer treatment ("pre-treatment") and after treatment at the follow-up 5–10 years later ("at follow-up").

We see from the figure that the IIEF scores are clustered up at the higher end of the scale before brachtherapy, with all men classified as potent (the vertical line in the middle of the graph represents the potency threshold of 11). After the therapy, however the distribution is much more spread out, with only 63 % (39/62) of the men potent and the other 37 % being classified as impotent, according to the index. Apparently, interference with erectile function is one of the "downsides" of brachytherapy.

In the next chapter we begin the study of inferential statistics. This body of techniques is concerned with two issues: testing a hypothesis about a population parameter and estimating the value of a population parameter. In the next chapter, we define what a hypothesis is and lay out the reasoning that leads to a test of its veracity. We will see that hypotheses are neither proved nor disproved. Rather, we will attempt to marshal evidence for the hypotheses that we believe to be true. And to the extent that they are continuously supported in ongoing studies, we will tend to accept them. To the extent that they are not supported in research, we will tend to doubt their veracity. Such is the nature of the scientific process.

Chapter 3
Testing a Hypothesis

This chapter introduces the reader to statistical inference, and in particular, the test of hypothesis. Inference refers to the idea that we will employ the sample data to make inferences about the population. A major means of making inferences is to pose a hypothesis about the population and then examine whether it is supported by one's sample data. There is an intricate set of cognitive steps involved in this process. Because reasoning is involved that may seem unfamiliar at first, we will proceed with caution. We begin with a simple and intuitive example of hypothesis testing to show the reader that he or she already employs such reasoning on a regular basis.

The Test of Hypothesis

The *test of hypothesis* is one of the major vehicles for assessing the truth or falsehood of a claim about the population. It is so important to the enterprise of inferential statistics that we will need to discuss it at length here. But, in fact, you already *know* how to perform a test of hypothesis. It involves reasoning that we all use all the time. Here's a simple, but instructional, example.

Let's Roll the Dice

Are you lucky with dice? Let's assume you are. So let's gamble with them. You and the first author of this primer, Al, will play the game. We each pony up a dollar and put it into the pot. Each of us has a die. We will each roll our die. Whoever has the highest number wins the pot. If there's a tie, we ante up again, the pot gets larger, and we keep rolling. What do you say?

Okay, here's how it goes. Al rolls a 6; you roll a 3. Then Al rolls a 6; you roll a 1. Then Al rolls a 6; you roll a 6. Then Al rolls a 6; you roll a 4. Then Al rolls a 5...

A. DeMaris and S.H. Selman, *Converting Data into Evidence: A Statistics Primer for the Medical Practitioner*, DOI 10.1007/978-1-4614-7792-1_3,
© Springer Science+Business Media New York 2013

wait a minute! By now we're betting you're stopping the game. You probably think Al's die is loaded. Why? Because with an honest die, you're thinking, there's no way Al would be rolling four sixes in a row. There's your test of hypothesis. You've already done it and made a decision. Let's look at the test again, but couched a little more formally.

Testing Whether Al's Die Is Loaded

What you think at this point is that Al's die is loaded. If it's an honest die, then the probability of a six coming up each time is *at most* $1/6 = 0.167$. So what you're saying is: since Al's die is loaded, the probability of his die showing a six is greater than $1/6$. This is a statement of the *research hypothesis*. The research hypothesis is *what you think is the case and what you will try to marshal evidence for*. A hypothesis is always a statement about a population parameter. In this case, the parameter is the probability that Al's die comes up 6. Let's denote that with P. The research hypothesis is then expressed as H_1: $P > 1/6$.

Now, you can't actually *see* that a die is loaded. So how are you going to show that the research hypothesis is right? The only way, really, is to show that the opposite hypothesis—that the die is honest—must be *wrong*. Because if the die is supposed to be honest, then you can calculate the probability of getting four sixes followed by a number that's not a six. And if that's very unlikely, then you've shown that the observed data—i.e., the five outcomes of Al's die rolls—are simply inconsistent with an honest die. That the die is honest is what's called the *null hypothesis*. The null hypothesis is *what we are typically trying to cast doubt upon*. In this example, it's H_0: $P \leq 1/6$.

Statement of Hypotheses

So, here are the two hypotheses:

H_0: $P \leq 1/6$
H_1: $P > 1/6$

Notice that the hypotheses are exhaustive. That is, all possible probabilities of a six coming up have been listed. And they're mutually exclusive. If one's right, the other's wrong, and vice versa.

Testing the Null Hypothesis

What we will test is the *plausibility of the null hypothesis*. To do that, we need a *test statistic*. In this case, the test statistic is the *number of sixes in Al's five die rolls*.

In general, the test statistic is a *sample measure whose probability of occurrence can be calculated if the null hypothesis is true.* Here's Al's sequence of roll outcomes, again.

AL: 6 6 6 6 O

Where the letter "O" here stands for "other than a six."

Since there are four sixes in 5 rolls, the test statistic is 4. Now we ask: what's the probability of getting 4 or more sixes in five die rolls with an honest die? And to give Al the greatest benefit of the doubt, we'll allow that the four sixes don't *have* to be the first four rolls, even though that's what his sequence was. But there are five different sequences that would have eventuated in four sixes. They are {6 6 6 6 O} (what he actually rolled); {O 6 6 6 6}; {6 O 6 6 6}; {6 6 O 6 6}; and {6 6 6 O 6}. Each such sequence has the following probability of occurrence, by the multiplication rule for probabilities:

$$\left(\frac{1}{6}\right)\left(\frac{1}{6}\right)\left(\frac{1}{6}\right)\left(\frac{1}{6}\right)\left(\frac{5}{6}\right) = 0.00064.$$

And since there are five such sequences that satisfy the event of getting four sixes, we multiply by 5 to get the probability of getting four sixes:

$$\text{Pr(4 sixes in 5 rolls with honest die)} = 5 \times \left(\frac{1}{6}\right)\left(\frac{1}{6}\right)\left(\frac{1}{6}\right)\left(\frac{1}{6}\right)\left(\frac{5}{6}\right) = 0.0032.$$

But we're not done. What we want is the probability of getting *at least* four sixes in five rolls. The reason is that *five* sixes is even more dramatic evidence against H_0, and that possibility has to be included, too. The probability of getting five sixes is:

$$\left(\frac{1}{6}\right)\left(\frac{1}{6}\right)\left(\frac{1}{6}\right)\left(\frac{1}{6}\right)\left(\frac{1}{6}\right) = 0.00013$$

In sum, the probability of getting four or more sixes in five tosses of an honest die is:

Pr (four or more sixes in five tosses of an honest die) = $0.0032 + 0.00013 = 0.00333$.

Making a Decision

The decision of whether or not to reject the null hypothesis hangs on this probability. It's so important that it's given a special name and notation in statistics: It's called *the p value*. (Notice that the lower-case "*p*" used here is different from the upper-case "*P*" used to represent the probability Al's die comes up 6.) It's defined as *the probability of getting sample results at least as unfavorable to H_0 as was observed if H_0 is true.* If it's too small, that means that *the observed result would be* *too unlikely under the null* ("under the null" means if the null hypothesis were true) *for the null hypothesis to be believable.* In this case, it's pretty small: there's only about a three in a thousand chance of getting at least four sixes in five rolls with an honest die. So you are right to reject the null hypothesis and conclude that Al's die is loaded.

Note: you haven't *proved* that his die is loaded. Even though unlikely, it is indeed *possible* to get four or more sixes in five tosses of an honest die. In fact, it would happen 0.333 % of the time. But which would you rather believe: you've just experienced a very, very rare event, or you're dealing with someone who's cheating? Knowing how much Al hates to lose money, we'd go with the latter.

"Statistically Significant" Results

Finally, you might ask: how small does the *p* value have to be for us to reject H_0? The answer is:

By convention, *when the p value is ≤ 0.05,* we reject the null hypothesis. The value of 0.05 is called the *alpha-level for the test*: it's the criterion probability we use for judging when the sample result is too unlikely to be believable. And when we reject H_0, we say that the test result is *statistically significant.* This terminology is so central to statistics that we'll say it again: When you reject the null hypothesis, you say, "The test result is statistically significant." In the dice example, this means that the probability of Al's die coming up 6 is greater than what was specified in the null hypothesis. In general, statistically significant results imply that the true value of the parameter of interest is *different* from what the null hypothesis posits.

What About Your Sequence of Die Rolls?

For comparative purposes let's consider the probability of *your* sequence of rolls. Now we didn't find out your last roll, but let's suppose it wasn't a 6. So your sequence was: 3 1 6 4 O.

With an honest die, you'd expect about one 6 to come up in five rolls. The probability of getting just one 6 is:

$$\text{Pr(1 six in 5 rolls with an honest die)} = 5 \times \left(\frac{1}{6}\right)\left(\frac{5}{6}\right)\left(\frac{5}{6}\right)\left(\frac{5}{6}\right)\left(\frac{5}{6}\right) = 0.402.$$

Or, we might ask: what's the probability of getting *at most* one six in five rolls of an honest die? Then we have to add the probability of getting no sixes, which is:

$$\left(\frac{5}{6}\right)\left(\frac{5}{6}\right)\left(\frac{5}{6}\right)\left(\frac{5}{6}\right)\left(\frac{5}{6}\right) = 0.402.$$

In sum, the probability of getting at most one six in five rolls of an honest die is $0.402 + 0.402 = 0.804$. At any rate, no one is going to accuse *you* of having a loaded die!

Large-Sample Test of Hypothesis About a Mean

Now let's apply what we just learned to understand a real statistical test. Recall the distribution of education in the 2002 GSS shown in the previous chapter. Recall that the mean is 13.36 and the standard deviation is 2.97. And the sample size is 2,753. We don't know what the mean education in the entire U.S. adult population was in that year, though. Although 13.36 is a good estimate, it's only an estimate. So suppose a firm was planning on creating a medical Web site in 2002 where people could read about health issues. They were planning on pitching it at a 12th-grade reading level because the company president insisted that the average person in the country had, at most, a high-school education. His vice president disagreed; he thought the average person had better than a high-school education. So let's do a test of hypothesis about the population mean of education to see who was right.

Assumptions for the Test

Every test is based on some assumptions or ground rules. If these assumptions are not satisfied, the test results may not be valid. For this test, which is called the *large-sample test of hypothesis about a population mean*, the assumptions are:

1. We have a random sample from the population. (We do, so that's satisfied.)
2. The variable in question is quantitative. (It's education, which is quantitative, so that's satisfied.)
3. The sample size is at least 30. (It's 2,753, so that's satisfied. Below we'll see why this last assumption is important.)

Statement of Hypotheses

Let μ represent mean education in the 2002 US adult population. Then the hypotheses are:

H_0: $\mu \leq 12$.
H_1: $\mu > 12$.

Before Going Further: The Sampling Distribution of a Sample Statistic

We must pause here. We need a test statistic that will allow us to find a *p* value for the test. That is, just as in the dice-rolling example above, we need to know the likelihood of getting the sample result we've observed (i.e., a mean education of 13.36) if the null hypothesis (that the population mean is less than or equal to 12) is true. However, to understand that test statistic and *p* value in this case, we need to discuss the single most important concept in all of inferential statistics: the sampling distribution of a sample statistic. Recall the dice example. Remember that we marshaled evidence for the research hypothesis (Al's die is loaded) by showing that the sample result (four or more sixes in five tosses) was implausible if the null was true.

In the current problem, the sample result is the sample mean, which is our best estimate of the population mean. We will marshal evidence for the research hypothesis that the population mean is greater than 12 by showing that, if the null is true (that the mean is, at most, 12), it is very unlikely to get a sample mean (13.36) that's at least as large as we've gotten. To know the likelihood of a particular sample mean when the population mean is a specific value, we use the *sampling distribution of the sample mean*. This is a *distribution of all of the sample means that would be found by infinite repetition of the sampling scheme*. That is, suppose that the GSS took a second random sample of 2,753 US adults in 2002, and then a third random sample of 2,753 adults in 2002, and so on, continuing until all possible nonredundant samples had been collected. Two samples are nonredundant provided that they do not contain the exact same population members. For each of these samples, mean education would be calculated. This (virtually) infinite collection of sample means would be the sampling distribution of the sample mean for this problem. If we have knowledge of the sampling distribution of the sample mean, we can figure out how likely it would be to get a sample mean of 13.36 or greater if the population mean is only 12.

Simple Example of a Sampling Distribution

To see a simple example of a sampling distribution, regard the following Table 3.1:

What we see first is a very small population consisting of five units, lettered A through E. For each unit, the variable *Y* has been measured and given a value. The population mean of *Y*, or μ (not shown), is 3 (as is easily verified). The population variance of *Y* (also not shown), which is given the symbol σ^2, is 2. How is the latter calculated? Since it's the population variance and not the sample estimate of the population variance, we divide by *N* rather than *N*−1:

$$\sigma^2 = \frac{(1-3)^2 + (2-3)^2 + (3-3)^2 + (4-3)^2 + (5-3)^2}{5} = \frac{10}{5} = 2.$$

Table 3.1 The sampling distribution for the sample mean and sample variance, Based on repeated sampling of size $N=3$ from a population with 5 units

Population Elements:

Case	Y
A	2
B	3
C	1
D	5
E	4

Sampling Distribution (for N = 3):

Sample	Members	Y	$\bar{y}$	Proportion	s^2	Proportion
1	A,B,C	2,3,1	2	.1	1	.3
2	A,B,D	2,3,5	3.33	.2	2.33	.4
3	A,B,E	2,3,4	3	.2	1	.3
4	A,C,D	2,1,5	2.67	.2	4.33	.2
5	A,C,E	2,1,4	2.33	.1	2.33	.4
6	A,D,E	2,5,4	3.67	.1	2.33	.4
7	B,C,D	3,1,5	3	.2	4	.1
8	B,C,E	3,1,4	2.67	.2	2.33	.4
9	B,D,E	3,5,4	4	.1	1	.3
10	C,D,E	1,5,4	3.33	.2	4.33	.2

Reprinted with permission of John Wiley & Sons, Inc., from DeMaris (2004)

Below that, we see 10 different nonredundant samples of size $N=3$ taken from this population. This is the total number of nonredundant random samples of size 3 that can be drawn from this population. Sampling is done here *without replacement*, which means that, for any given sample, once a unit is drawn into the sample, it's no longer available to be drawn again into that same sample.

For each sample, two statistics have been calculated: the sample mean, denoted "$\bar{y}$" (and pronounced "y-bar"), and the sample variance (s^2, as before). The "Proportion" columns show the proportionate representation of each sample mean or variance in the collection. So the sample mean of 2 occurs just once, which is 10 % of the time, whereas the sample mean of 2.67 occurs twice, or 20 % of the time, and so forth.

We focus on the sample mean first. Notice that there is some variability in the sample means. They range from 2 to 4 in value. That is, they bracket the population mean of 3. Sample means that are closer to 3—such as 2.67, 3, and 3.33—are more likely to be observed than those that are farther away from it (such as 2, 2.33, 3.67, or 4). So even in this very simplified example, you're more likely to get a sample mean that's close to the population mean than one that's farther away, when you take a random sample.

The column of means and its associated Proportion column together constitute the *sampling distribution of the sample mean*. The sampling distribution of the sample mean is a *probability distribution*. It shows all possible sample means that could be observed using a given sample size, along with their probabilities of being observed. Moreover, this distribution itself has a mean and a standard deviation. Let's find the mean of the sampling distribution of sample means:

$$\text{Mean } (\bar{y}) = \frac{2 + 3.33 + 3 + 2.67 + 2.33 + 3.67 + 3 + 2.67 + 4 + 3.33}{10} = 3.$$

Notice that this is exactly the same as the population mean of Y that we're trying to estimate using the sample mean. This phenomenon is not a coincidence. It turns out that the mean of the sampling distribution of sample means is always equal to the population mean you're trying to estimate. For this reason, we say that the sample mean is an *unbiased* estimator of the population mean. "Unbiased" simply means that the average value of the sample statistic (averaging over its sampling distribution) is equal to the population parameter it's meant to estimate.

We can also calculate the standard deviation of the sample means. First, we calculate the sum of squared deviations of each sample mean from the mean of the sample means:

$$\begin{aligned}
\text{Sum of squared deviations} = &(2-3)^2 + (3.33-3)^2 + (3-3)^2 + (2.67-3)^2 \\
&+ (2.33-3)^2 + (3.67-3)^2 + (3-3)^2 \\
&+ (2.67-3)^2 + (4-3)^2 + (3.33-3)^2 = 3.3334.
\end{aligned}$$

Now, to get the variance of the sample means, we divide the sum of squares by 10 (not 9, since it's not an estimator of the variance of sample means, rather it *is* the variance of the sample means):

$$\text{Variance}(\bar{y}) = \frac{0.3334}{10} = 0.33334.$$

Finally, to get the standard deviation of sample means, we take the square root of 0.33334 to get 0.577.

The standard deviation of sample means is called the *standard error of the mean*, since it indicates the average amount of error one incurs in using the sample mean to estimate the population mean. Finally, we should note that a similar set of

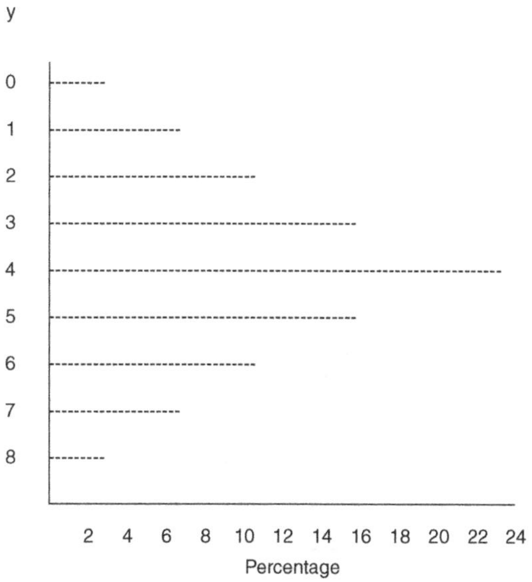

y		Freq	Cum. Freq	Percent	Cum. Percent
0	--------	1	1	3.45	3.45
1	------------------	2	3	6.90	10.34
2	--------------------------------	3	6	10.34	20.69
3	---	5	11	17.24	37.93
4	---	7	18	24.14	62.07
5	---	5	23	17.24	79.31
6	--------------------------------	3	26	10.34	89.66
7	------------------	2	28	6.90	96.55
8	--------	1	29	3.45	100.00

```
        2   4   6   8  10  12  14  16  18  20  22  24
                       Percentage
```

Fig. 3.1 Population distribution for the variable $Y = \text{PSA}$ of men on Johnson's Island

operations would also give us the mean and standard error of the sample variances from these ten samples. Bottom line: every sample statistic has a sampling distribution, and that distribution has a mean and a standard deviation. The standard deviation of a sampling distribution is called a *standard error*, to distinguish it from the ordinary standard deviation of just any variable.

A More Elaborate Example

The example of sampling distributions above is rudimentary and serves only to introduce the idea. Let's take a look at a slightly more elaborate example to get a better sense of what the sampling distribution of the sample mean will look like with a larger population.

Johnson's Island is a tiny atoll in the Pacific Ocean. There is a population of men who live on it to maintain critical navigation equipment for transoceanic travel. Suppose the population of adult males on Johnson's Island consists of 29 males. A urologist is interested in estimating mean PSA level for this population. So he decides to take a random sample of five men, measure their PSA, and then use the sample mean as his estimate of the population mean. What does the sampling distribution of the sample mean look like for this population and this sample size?

Let $y =$ the variable "PSA." First, here is the distribution of y for the 29 men in the population (Fig. 3.1):

This is a horizontal bar chart. The values of Y form the rows of the chart. The numbers of men with each different value of PSA are represented by the lengths of

Percentage

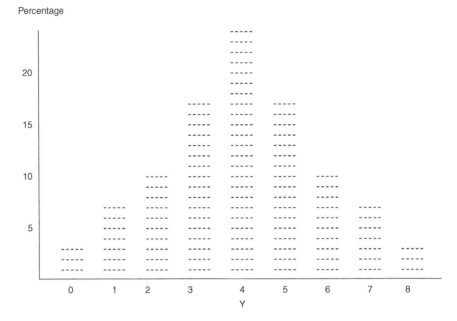

Fig. 3.2 Population distribution for the variable $Y=$ PSA of men on Johnson's Island: Rotated counterclockwise

the bars. These numbers are also given in the "Freq" column. For example, one man has a PSA of 0, five men have a PSA of 3, seven men have a PSA of 4, and so forth. As we can see from the Y values, PSA levels in the population range from 0 to 8. Mean PSA in the population is 4 and the standard deviation of PSA for the population is $\sigma = 1.875$ (not shown). Let's look at this distribution again, but rotated 90° counterclockwise (Fig. 3.2).

This is a vertical bar chart. The values of PSA are on the horizontal axis. The heights of the "bars" (represented with layers of dashes) represent the percentages of men having each value of PSA. Notice that this distribution somewhat resembles a normal distribution, with values bunching up between 3 and 5, and then fewer men having values of 0–2 or 6–8.

Next, we present the sampling distribution of the sample mean for this population and a sample size of 5. We will see a depiction of all possible sample means we could get when sampling from this population. Here sampling is done, again, without replacement. This means that every sample is unique in not having the exact same population members as any other sample. This distribution is shown in Fig. 3.3.

Here, we see that the sample means range from 1.2 to 6.8. We also see that the total number of sample means in the sampling distribution is 118,755 (given at the bottom of the "Cum. Freq" column). The "Freq" column shows that very few sample means are as low as 1.2 or as high as 6.8. In fact, only three samples each have

Distribution of the Sample Mean   for n = 5:

ybar		Freq	Cum. Freq	Percent	Cum. Percent
1.2		3	3	0.00	0.00
1.4		17	20	0.01	0.02
1.6		62	82	0.05	0.07
1.8	-	172	254	0.14	0.21
2.0	--	413	667	0.35	0.56
2.2	----	834	1501	0.70	1.26
2.4	------	1529	3030	1.29	2.55
2.6	-----------	2541	5571	2.14	4.69
2.8	----------------	3899	9470	3.28	7.97
3.0	----------------------	5520	14990	4.65	12.62
3.2	------------------------------	7316	22306	6.16	18.78
3.4	-------------------------------------	9056	31362	7.63	26.41
3.6	---	10545	41907	8.88	35.29
3.8	--	11526	53433	9.71	44.99
4.0	--	11889	65322	10.01	55.01
4.2	--	11526	76848	9.71	64.71
4.4	---	10545	87393	8.88	73.59
4.6	-------------------------------------	9056	96449	7.63	81.22
4.8	------------------------------	7316	103765	6.16	87.38
5.0	----------------------	5520	109285	4.65	92.03
5.2	----------------	3899	113184	3.28	95.31
5.4	-----------	2541	115725	2.14	97.45
5.6	------	1529	117254	1.29	98.74
5.8	----	834	118088	0.70	99.44
6.0	--	413	118501	0.35	99.79
6.2	-	172	118673	0.14	99.93
6.4		62	118735	0.05	99.98
6.6		17	118752	0.01	100.00
6.8		3	118755	0.00	100.00

```
        1   2   3   4   5   6   7   8   9   10

            Percentage
```

Fig. 3.3 Sampling distribution of the sample mean of PSA from the population of PSA values on Johnson's Island for $n=5$

means that are this far from the population mean of PSA, which we know is 4. The most common sample mean, as shown by the "Freq" column, is the value 4, with a "Freq" of 11,889. That is, the most likely value of a sample mean when sampling randomly from this population is the value 4, which is the same as the population mean of Y. Once again, let's see this distribution when rotated counterclockwise 90°. Figure 3.4 shows the result.

Notice that this distribution very much resembles a normal distribution. This is not a coincidence, as we will see with the important theorem *Central Limit Theorem* (CLT) presented below. Notice also that the highest "bar" in this distribution is for the value 4.0. In fact, the average of all these sample means is 4.0, the same as the population mean of Y. The standard deviation of all these sample means is 0.8. This is also equal to σ, the population standard deviation of Y, divided by the square root of the sample size. That is, $\dfrac{\sigma}{\sqrt{n}} = \dfrac{1.875}{\sqrt{5}} = 0.8$. This is also not a coincidence, as the CLT tells us, below.

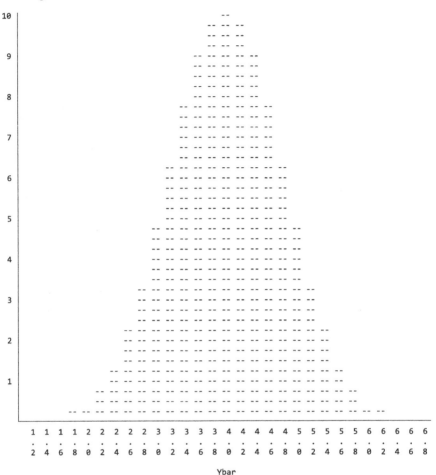

Fig. 3.4 Sampling distribution of the sample mean of PSA from the population of PSA Values on Johnson's Island for $n = 5$: Rotated counterclockwise

Sampling Distribution of the Mean for the Large-Sample Test of Hypothesis

Okay, back to our test of hypothesis about mean education. We need the sampling distribution of the sample mean for that problem, which you recall is based on a sample size of 2,753. We certainly don't want to try to generate all possible samples like we did in Table 3.1 or the Johnson's Island example above! Fortunately, we don't have to. There is a statistical theorem called the CLT that tells us what that sampling distribution looks like.

The Central Limit Theorem

There are two corollaries to the CLT. The first is that if a variable Y is normally distributed in the population, and we are using random sampling, then the sampling distribution of the sample mean, $\bar{y}$, is a *normal* distribution, regardless how large or small the sample size is. Moreover, the mean of the sampling distribution is μ, the population mean of Y. And the standard deviation of the sampling distribution of $\bar{y}$ (i.e., the "standard error" of the sample mean) is equal to $\dfrac{\sigma}{\sqrt{n}}$, where σ is the standard deviation of Y in the population. As we saw in the Johnson's Island example, the distribution of the 29 values of Y in the "population" kind of resembled a normal distribution, and the resulting sampling distribution of $\bar{y}$ looked *very* much like a normal distribution, even with a small sample of size 5.

The second corollary of the CLT is much more important than the first. Typically, the distribution of Y in the population is not at all normal. Nevertheless, the CLT says that as long as you're using random sampling, and the sample size is large, the sampling distribution of the sample mean is still a *normal distribution*. The mean of that distribution is μ, the population mean that we are trying to test a hypothesis about. And the standard error of the mean (i.e., the standard deviation of the sampling distribution of $\bar{y}$) is $\dfrac{\sigma}{\sqrt{n}}$. This is really a remarkable result. It means that as long as we have a large sample, it does not matter how the variable in question is distributed in the population. We know that the sampling distribution of the sample mean is normal in shape, centered over the population mean of the variable in question, and with a standard deviation that has a simple formula ($\dfrac{\sigma}{\sqrt{n}}$). How large is a "large" sample? It turns out that if n is ≥ 30, that's large enough.

In the education example, the population mean in question is mean education for US adults in 2002. The sample size is 2,753—plenty large. By the CLT, then, we know that the sampling distribution of the sample mean of education is normal. Moreover, the standard deviation, or standard error, of this sampling distribution is equal to $\dfrac{\sigma}{\sqrt{2753}}$. Now, we don't know σ, but we can substitute the sample standard deviation of education into this formula in place of it. It turns out that this works just as well. The sample standard deviation of education in the GSS is 2.97. Thus, the estimate of the standard error of the sample mean is:

$$\text{Standard error of } \bar{y} = \frac{2.97}{\sqrt{2753}} = 0.057.$$

Test Statistic and P-Value

So here's the deal: to accomplish our test of hypothesis, we need to find the probability of getting a sample mean of at least 13.36 if the population mean is 12. Now we know that the sample mean has a normal distribution centered over μ. So let's assume μ is 12. The test is always conducted "under the null hypothesis," meaning, by assuming the null hypothesis is true. The reason is that it is the plausibility of H_0 that is actually being tested. To find the p value that determines the test's outcome, we have to find the probability of getting a sample mean of 13.36 or greater when sampling from a normal distribution whose mean is 12. Regard the normal distribution in Fig. 2.5 from the previous chapter again. Imagine that, instead of 0, it's centered over 12. Then 13.36 is way over in the right tail of the distribution. To find the probability associated with all values ≥ 13.36, we have to find the area in that part of the tail. And there is a table that lets us do this, which is found in most statistics texts. It tells the probability of being a particular number of standard deviations away from the mean of a normal distribution. How many standard deviations (of the sampling distribution of $\bar{y}$) away from 12 is 13.36? That's easy, it's:

$$z = \frac{13.36 - 12}{0.057} = 23.9 \text{ standard deviations above 12.}$$

Using the table, we find that the probability of being that far above μ on a normal distribution is <0.00001. Therefore, the p value is expressed as "$p < 0.00001$."

Summary

Our test statistic is the "z" calculation above. It converts an observed sample mean into its distance from the null-hypothesized population mean. So, like the dice-rolling example, it tells us how much of a discrepancy there is between what we'd expect to see if the null hypothesis is true—which is a sample mean of 12—from what we actually observed—which is a sample mean of 13.36. The p value in this case is so small we're just expressing it as "<0.00001." But it's easy to see that we will reject the null hypothesis here in favor of the research hypothesis. That is, we conclude that the mean education of adults in the US in 2002 was greater than just 12 years of schooling.

A few closing comments are in order. First, what you'd "expect" to see if the null hypothesis is true is statistical lingo. In statistics, the "expected value" of anything is its population mean. The expected value of the sample mean is the mean of its sampling distribution, and this is what you'd "expect" to see in the sense that it's the average value of the sample mean. So it's the sample mean you'd get, on average, when taking a sample from the population. So if the null were true in this example, you'd "expect" the sample mean to be 12. Second, there is a lesson to take away from this test about the construction of a test statistic. All test statistics in statistics measure *how much of a discrepancy there is between what you actually observe in a sample and what you'd expect to see if the null is true*. Hypothesis testing is not the only way to make inferences about the population. Instead, we can just try to estimate the value of the parameter in question. However, this estimate needs to be qualified by a "margin of error," since it is subject to sampling variability. The next chapter details this approach, along with additional topics pertinent to statistical inference.

Chapter 4
Additional Inferential Procedures

Confidence Intervals and the T Test

In this chapter we discuss the confidence interval. This is an interval of numbers that, we are very confident, contains the parameter of interest. Such intervals are very useful when our interest is in what the value of the parameter actually is, rather than just whether our hypothesis about it is or is not supported. After that, we revisit hypothesis testing with a more elaborate test in which we test whether two means in the population are the same. Following this, we consider the issue of statistical power in hypothesis testing. Power is a very important consideration, particularly when researchers are deciding how large a sample they need to collect in order to effectively answer their research questions.

Confidence Intervals

We continue with the example of testing whether mean education in the USA was ≤ 12 years, from the previous chapter. Testing hypotheses is one way to conduct inferences. However, it doesn't really tell us what the actual parameter value is. It just tells us we can reject that it is in some range of values (e.g., ≤ 12) and accept that it is in some other range of values (e.g., >12). But this isn't all that informative. So is it, say, 12.1? 12.2? 13? 14? 15? In this example, where our interest centers on a single population mean, it's much more useful to try to pin down its actual value with some precision. For this purpose, we typically use a *confidence interval*. This is an interval of numbers that, we are very confident, contains the true parameter value. It is based, again, on the sampling distribution of a statistic. Recall that the sample mean of education is normally distributed, with a standard error of 0.057. And the true population mean is smack in the middle of the distribution. Now, in conducting the test of hypothesis, we assumed that μ was 12. For the confidence

A. DeMaris and S.H. Selman, *Converting Data into Evidence: A Statistics Primer for the Medical Practitioner*, DOI 10.1007/978-1-4614-7792-1_4, © Springer Science+Business Media New York 2013

interval we're not going to assume anything about μ. Rather, we take advantage of the fact that 95 % of all sample means of education are within 1.96 standard errors of μ (as noted above). To form a 95 % confidence interval for μ, we simply add and subtract 1.96 standard errors from the sample mean. Hence

95% Confidence interval for mean education $= 13.36 \pm 1.96(0.057) = (13.25, 13.47)$.

We say, then, that we are 95 % confident that mean education of all US noninstitutionalized adults in 2002 was between 13.25 and 13.47 years of schooling. This works because 95 % of the time with a random sample of 2,753 cases from this population, such an interval will contain the true value of μ. Why does this work? Remember that the sample mean is normally distributed. The center of this distribution is the population mean that we are trying to estimate. Our particular sample mean is one of the means in this distribution. We don't know whether it is above the center of the distribution or below the center of the distribution. But if we attach an interval of numbers that is equal to 1.96 standard errors of the sample mean to either "side" of our sample mean, there is only a 5 % chance that the resulting interval will not contain the population mean.

We'll use an analogy to drive home the point. Suppose you're in a pitch-dark closet. It's very small. There's a light switch on the wall, but you don't know if it's on the wall to your left or on the wall to your right. But you also know that only 2.5 % of the closet is too far from the switch for it to be reached by hand from anywhere in the closet. Your arm is exactly 1.96 feet long. So if the switch is on the left wall, and you reach for it with your left hand, there's only a 2.5 % chance you won't reach it. And if the switch is on the right wall, and you reach for it with your right hand, there's only a 2.5 % chance that you won't reach it. So, altogether, if you just reach out both hands, there's only a 5 % chance you won't reach the light switch.[1] Which means you're 95 % confident that reaching out both hands will let you turn on the light.

In sum, confidence intervals should be seen as a useful supplement to the test of hypothesis. In particular, if the result is significant, we may want to follow up with a confidence interval to pin down the value of the parameter of interest.

Testing the Difference Between Two Means: The T *Test*

Hypothesis tests are typically reserved for analyzing the relationship between at least two variables. Recall the diet-study data in Table 2.1. We're interested in

---

[1] By rules of probability: For two mutually exclusive events A and B, $\Pr(A \text{ or } B) = \Pr(A) + \Pr(B)$. So let $A =$ you're to the right of the light switch and too far away, and $B =$ you're to the left of the light switch and too far away. Then $\Pr(\text{you won't reach the switch}) = \Pr(\text{you're right of the switch and too far away } or \text{ you're left of the switch and too far away}) = \Pr(\text{you're right of the switch and too far away}) + \Pr(\text{you're left of the switch and too far away}) = 0.025 + 0.025 = 0.05$. QED.

whether a treatment variable, diet, affects a response variable (also called a "study endpoint"), PSA level. We will use these data to test our hypothesis about the deleterious effect of a steak diet on PSA. For the moment we'll confine our attention to the first two columns (we'll leave the men on a vegetarian diet for a later test). In this case, our research hypothesis is a diet rich in red meat results in an elevated PSA, compared to a balanced diet. To show support for this, we also tender the opposite proposition, the *null* hypothesis: a diet rich in red meat will, at most, result in the same PSA level as a balanced diet (but could also be associated with a lower PSA level). As before, the way we will try to marshal support for the research hypothesis is to show that the data are inconsistent with the null hypothesis.

Statement of Hypotheses

Hypotheses refer to what is true in the population. We assume there are two subpopulations: the population of men on the control diet, group 1, and the population of men on the steak diet, group 2. Let the mean PSA levels for these two subpopulations be denoted μ_1 and μ_2, respectively. The standard deviation of PSA in each subpopulation is assumed, for this particular test, to be the same, and is denoted σ. The hypotheses are expressed as follows:

Null hypothesis: $\mu_2 \leq \mu_1$.
Research hypothesis: $\mu_2 > \mu_1$.

But it is more informative to express both hypotheses in terms of one parameter, $\mu_2 - \mu_1$, the *mean difference* between the groups. In particular:

Null hypothesis: $\mu_2 - \mu_1 \leq 0$.
Research hypothesis: $\mu_2 - \mu_1 > 0$.

Sample Information and the Sampling Distribution

Now, the sample data in Table 2.1 provide us with evidence about this parameter, and, therefore, these hypotheses. The mean PSA for the steak group is 4.52 (as we calculated before) and for the control group it's 3.77. The sample mean difference is therefore $4.52 - 3.77 = 0.75$. If the null hypothesis is true, then this difference is supposed to be zero in the population (this would be the maximum difference that would obtain under the null hypothesis).

As before, the CLT tells us what the sampling distribution of mean differences looks like. If PSA levels are normally distributed in each subpopulation (control diet vs. steak diet), and we are using random sampling, then the sample mean differences have a *normal distribution* centered over the parameter of interest—which is the population mean difference in question. In particular, if the null hypothesis is true, the mean of the sampling distribution is zero, and it looks like the normal distribution in Fig. 2.5. For this reason, we can figure out how probable it is to get a mean difference of 0.75 or more if the population mean difference is, at most, zero.

The probability in question is based on a test called the *independent-samples, pooled-variance t test for a difference of means*. Often it's just called the "*t* test" for short. The reader should be aware, however, that there is not just one *t* test, but rather several different ones, so named because of their reliance on the *t* distribution (also shown in Fig. 2.5). The assumptions for the independent-samples, pooled-variance *t* test for a difference of means are:

Assumptions for the **T** *Test*

1. We have a random sample from each subpopulation. (We do.)
2. The study endpoint is a quantitative variable. (It's PSA level, so it is.)
3. The study endpoint is normally distributed in each subpopulation. (Let's assume it is.)
4. The variance of the study endpoint (i.e., PSA) is the same in each subpopulation. It is denoted σ^2. (Let's assume it is the same.)

Computation of the Test Statistic

The test is computed as follows. Let $\bar{x}_1$ be the sample mean PSA level for the control group. Its value is 3.77. Let $\bar{x}_2$ be the sample mean PSA level for the Steak group. Its value is 4.52. Let s_1 be the standard deviation of PSA in the control group. Its value is 1.38. Let s_2 be the standard deviation of PSA in the Steak group. From our earlier calculation, its value is 2.33. Let n be sample size in each group (in this case, n is 6). Then the formula for the t test statistic is (this form of the formula applies only with equal n in each group)

$$t = \frac{\bar{x}_2 - \bar{x}_1}{s_p \sqrt{\dfrac{2}{n}}} \qquad (4.1)$$

where s_p is the square root of the average of s_1^2 and s_2^2, and is therefore an estimate of the common subpopulation standard deviation of PSA, σ.

In the current problem, s_p is

$$s_p = \sqrt{\frac{1.38^2 + 2.33^2}{2}} = 1.91.$$

And, therefore, the calculated test statistic in the diet example is

$$t = \frac{4.52 - 3.77}{1.91\sqrt{\dfrac{2}{6}}} = 0.68. \tag{4.2}$$

Finding the **P** *Value*

If the null hypothesis is true, this statistic has a *t distribution* with, in this case, 10 degrees of freedom (df). That is, the sampling distribution of "*t*" here is *t* shaped, rather than normal (see Fig. 2.5 for the difference between the normal and *t* distributions). As is always true, the test statistic's value tells us *how much discrepancy there is between what we observe in the sample and what we would expect to observe if the null hypothesis were true*. So the question is: how likely is a discrepancy this large or larger? And the answer can be found by looking up the probability of getting a *t* value of 0.68 or larger in a *t* distribution with 10 df. This will be the *p* value for the test. A *t* table is found in most statistics texts. The *p* value turns out to be 0.26, which is larger than 0.05. Therefore, we fail to reject the null hypothesis here. There is not enough evidence to suggest that a meat diet leads to a higher PSA, on average, compared to a balanced diet.

One-Tailed vs. Two-Tailed Tests

The test we've just conducted is called a *one-tailed test*. The reason is that we look up the probability in only one tail of the *t* distribution (the right tail, in this case). That's because our research hypothesis is directional: if there's any difference in the groups, we're confident the Steak group will have a higher mean PSA. Most of the time, however, we're not so confident in the direction the results are going to take. And we do a *two-tailed test*. Formally, this means that our research hypothesis is bidirectional; that is, we entertain the possibility that the mean difference can be either positive or negative. With a two-tailed test, we have to double the *p* value that we'd get if it were one tailed. So if we were doing a two-tailed test in the diet example, the *p* value would be reported as 2(0.26)=0.52. Note that even though the formal research hypothesis might be bidirectional, if the result is significant, we still make a *directional conclusion*. That is, if the diet example were a two-tailed test and it had been significant, we would not just conclude that mean PSA levels were different for the groups. We'd conclude that a meat diet *raises* average PSA, since that's what the sample results are indicating.

Summary: Hypothesis Testing

At this point let's summarize all the steps in the test of hypothesis, using the diet study as our example. All tests of hypothesis follow the following format. The five steps in a test of hypothesis are as follows:

1. *State assumptions required for the test.* All tests rest on some assumptions, or ground rules. If these are not satisfied, the validity of the test and its conclusions may be in jeopardy. For our test, the assumptions are (a) that we have taken random samples of men from each diet "subpopulation," (b) that PSA is normally distributed in each subpopulation, (c) that the variance (or standard deviation) of PSA is the same in each subpopulation, and (d) that the study endpoint is quantitative. Some commentary is in order. The normal distribution assumption is less important if n is large in each group. For example, if n is 30 or more in each group, the assumption can be violated without invalidating the test. In the case of PSA, sample sizes of 30 or more in each group would be important, because PSA values tend to be right skewed rather than normally distributed. The reason why large ns are critical is that the CLT tells us that the sampling distribution of the mean difference (i.e., $\bar{x}_2 - \bar{x}_1$) will be approximately normal if the ns are large enough. This means that the test statistic, t, will have the t sampling distribution, and the test will still be valid despite the nonnormality of PSA in each group. The equal-variance assumption is also unimportant when n is exactly the same in each group, as it is in the example. If the test is done as a two-tailed test, it is particularly *robust*. Robust procedures are those that still give valid results even when their assumptions are violated. If one is especially concerned about the assumptions being satisfied, an alternative is to use a *nonparametric* test such as the *Wilcoxon test* or the *Mann–Whitney test*. Nonparameteric tests make no assumptions about the distribution of one's data in the population. They are especially useful for small samples and 1-sided tests, or cases in which the subpopulation distributions on the variable of interest are highly skewed. Nonparametric tests, like all tests, however, involve a test statistic and p value. These are interpreted in the same manner as the ones above. (The next chapter illustrates the Wilcoxon Rank Sum Test, a nonparametric alternative to the t test shown here.) One might ask why we don't just always use nonparameteric tests, if they don't rely on as many assumptions. The reason is that they are not as *powerful* as the parametric tests we've demonstrated here. Power will be discussed below.
2. *State the hypotheses.* The hypotheses for the diet example are shown above. There will always be a null hypothesis and a research hypothesis.
3. *Compute the test statistic.* Recall that a test statistic, in general, tells us how much discrepancy there is between what we observe in the sample and what we would expect to observe if the null hypothesis were true. And one other thing: it has to have a *known probability distribution* (e.g., normal distribution, t distribution, etc.) under the null. In the diet example, the formula and computation for the independent-samples pooled-variance t test are shown above. And the test statistic has a t distribution under the null.

4. *State the p value.* If calculating a test by hand, there are tables available that give the probabilities (i.e., the *p* values) associated with test-statistic values. If using software, the *p* value will be reported in the output.
5. *Make a decision.* If $p \leq 0.05$, reject the null and accept the research hypothesis. If $p > 0.05$, do not reject the null hypothesis.

Decision Errors and the Power of the Test

In any test of hypothesis there is a chance that we will make a decision error. For example, if we are using an alpha level of 0.05, then there is a 0.05, or 5 %, chance that we will reject a true null hypothesis. Why? Because 5 % of the time, when the null is true, you can get sample results that are far enough from what you'd expect that you'll end up rejecting the null. This type of error is called a *Type I error.* The chance of a Type I error is equal to the alpha level for the test. If you don't want to take that much of a chance on rejecting a true null, you can pick a lower alpha level to use, such as 0.02, 0.01, 0.001, and so forth. On the other hand, there is also a chance that you will fail to reject a false null. This is called a *Type II error.* We cannot specify ahead of time what its probability is because it depends upon what the true value of the parameter is. But whatever this probability, if you subtract it from 1.0, you have what's called the *power of the test.* The power of the test is the *probability that you will reject a false null hypothesis using a particular test with a particular sample size.* In other words, the power of the test is the probability that, if the null hypothesis is wrong, your test will lead you to reject it. And, as with a Type II error, it depends on the true value of the parameter. For example, the parameter in the *t* test for the diet study is the mean difference in PSA between steak- and balanced-diet groups. All else equal, we want as much power as possible. That is, we want to know that if the null hypothesis is really false, our test statistic will lead to its rejection. Power values of 0.80 or higher are considered optimum in medical research, as the applications below illustrate. Power becomes especially relevant when we fail to reject H_0. Then the question is: is the null really true, or did we simply not have enough power in our analysis to detect that it was false?

Power of the T *Test in the Diet Example*

In the diet study, we were not able to reject the null hypothesis of no mean difference. Most likely this is due to low power. The null may well be false but we just don't have enough power to detect it. Let's calculate the power of our test in this example. However, we will make an assumption to simplify the calculations (since power calculations can get quite complicated). Let's assume that σ, the standard deviation of PSA that characterizes both populations of men, is a known quantity. Normally that wouldn't be the case; we'd have to estimate it with sample data. But

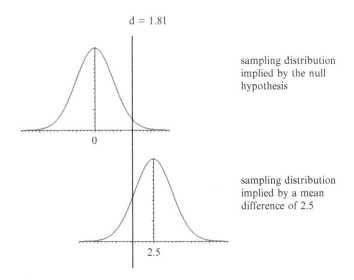

d = 1.81

sampling distribution
implied by the null
hypothesis

0

sampling distribution
implied by a mean
difference of 2.5

2.5

Fig. 4.1 The power of the T test for a difference of means

now let's just suppose we know its value. Further, we'll assume that it is equal to
1.91, the same as s_p, its estimated value above. What this means is that, instead of a
t distribution, our "t" statistic in (4.1) above actually has a *normal distribution*. And
the normal distribution is much easier to use for power calculations. To calculate
power, we first have to specify what the true parameter value is. So let's say the true
mean difference in PSA between groups is 2.5. This would be a clinically meaningful difference. So, what is the power of our test if the mean difference in the population is really 2.5?

Figure 4.1 depicts the scenario. Recall that every sample statistic has a sampling
distribution. The sample mean difference between diet groups is also a sample statistic. Therefore it, too, has a sampling distribution. Under the assumptions for the
test, it's a normal distribution. And its standard deviation, or standard error, is the
denominator of (4.2). That is, it is $1.91\sqrt{\dfrac{2}{6}} = 1.1$. What we see in Fig. 4.1 are two
sampling distributions for the sample mean difference, a top one and a bottom one.
The top one is the sampling distribution of the sample mean difference if the null
hypothesis is true. It's centered over zero. This is the sampling distribution that
we're basing our test and our conclusion on. The bottom distribution is the sampling
distribution of the sample mean difference if the research hypothesis is true, and, in
particular, if the mean difference is actually 2.5. Notice that this distribution is
therefore centered over 2.5 and has the same standard error.

Now we ask: what would cause us to reject the null? We will reject the null if our
p value is 0.05 or less. Using a table for the normal distribution, we find that we
would need a test statistic value of 1.645 or more to reject the null at a p value of
0.05. This means that we would need a sample mean difference that is at least 1.645
standard errors above zero before we could reject the null hypothesis. So we would

need a sample mean difference of at least $(1.645)(1.1) = 1.81$. This value is labeled "d" in the figure and is indicated by the vertical bar that goes through the right tail of the top distribution. The area to the right of that bar is 0.05, which is, incidentally, the probability of making a Type I error in this test.

However, the vertical bar goes through the bottom distribution, too, but it's left of the mean of that distribution. That is, a mean difference of 1.81 is below the center of that distribution, which is 2.5. To calculate our power, we ask: what is the probability of getting a sample mean difference of at least 1.81 *if the population mean difference is really 2.5*? Notice that the bottom sampling distribution is now what is determining how large a sample mean difference we would actually observe. For a normal distribution with mean 2.5 and standard deviation of 1.1, the probability of a sample mean difference of 1.81 or higher is the area to the right of the vertical line in the bottom distribution. Using a table for the normal distribution, we would find that it's 0.73. Hence 0.73 is the power of the test. Power should be at least around 0.70 or more to be considered minimally acceptable.

Now, if the true mean difference is 4.0, a very clinically significant amount, then our power increases to 0.98. That sounds pretty good. But what if the true mean difference is only, say, 1.0? Then our power is only 0.22. In this case, the null hypothesis would be patently false, but there's only a 22 % chance that our test will detect it. All else equal, power increases with the discrepancy between the true value of the parameter and what it is hypothesized to be under the null. And all else equal, power increases with sample size. Power considerations are extremely important when seeking external funding for research. In that case, power analyses are used to justify the expense of collecting a large enough sample to have adequate power for one's tests.

T *Tests for the GSS Data*

As another example of testing for a mean difference, let's do a *t* test using the 2002 GSS. Gender differences are always of interest. One question is whether men or women are higher in physician stewardship. At first glance, you might say women. After all, it's the stuff of standup comedy that men refuse to ask for directions when driving, right? So it would be reasonable that they would be more prone to want to ferret out health information on their own, rather than just listen to their doctor, compared to women. On the other hand, women are more health-conscious than men. They are more aware of symptoms of ill health, and they are more likely to seek medical attention when ill. Therefore they might be more proactive about obtaining their own information about health problems than men are.

Let's play it safe, then, and do a two-tailed test. This time, let group 0 be males and group 1 be females. Then μ_0 is mean physician stewardship in the 2002 population of US males and μ_1 is mean physician stewardship in the population of US females. The hypotheses are as follows:

H_0: $\mu_0 = \mu_1$.
H_1: $\mu_0 \neq \mu_1$.

Table 4.1 Stata output for the test for a gender difference in physician stewardship

```
                       Two-sample t test with equal variances
--------------------------------------------------------------------------
  Group |    Obs        Mean   Std. Err.    Std.Dev.  [95% Conf. Interval]
--------+-----------------------------------------------------------------
      0 |   1222    3.484452    .0511729    1.788855  3.384055    3.584848
      1 |   1524    3.051837    .0465102    1.815687  2.960606    3.143068
--------+-----------------------------------------------------------------
combined|   2746    3.244355    .0346596    1.816243  3.176394    3.312317
--------+-----------------------------------------------------------------
   diff |              .4326144    .0692644              .2967989     .56843
--------------------------------------------------------------------------
   diff = mean(0) - mean(1)                                  t =    6.2458
Ho: diff = 0                                   degrees of freedom =      2744

   Ha: diff < 0                  Ha: diff != 0                  Ha: diff > 0
Pr(T < t) = 1.0000        Pr(|T| > |t|) = 0.0000        Pr(T > t) = 0.0000
```

Table 4.1 presents the software output showing the test results, from a popular statistical software program called Stata.

In this output, "Obs" is the sample size in each group. The mean for physician stewardship for each group (the groups are labeled "0" for males and "1" for females) is shown under "Mean," as is the difference between the means (shown as "diff"). The mean difference is 0.433. This is computed by subtracting the female mean from the male mean. We see that it is actually males who are higher in physician stewardship. That is, they are more willing to rely on the physician's knowledge than women are. Is this a significant difference? At the bottom of the table we see that it is. The two-tailed p value is shown as "$P(|T| > |t|) = 0.0000$." This doesn't mean that the p value is literally zero. Rather, the p value is <0.00005. If it had been 0.00005, it would have been rounded up to 0.0001. Notice also that at the far right in the "diff" row there is a 95 % confidence interval given for the mean gender difference in physician stewardship. Hence, we can be 95 % confident that the mean difference is between about 0.297 and 0.568.

Comments About Statistical Tests

At this point in the primer, we've covered some statistical basics. Topics covered include samples and populations, causality and latent selection factors, describing variables and their distributions in samples, ways of summarizing data, describing population distributions, understanding the sampling distribution, and statistical inferences via tests of hypothesis and confidence intervals. There are some additional nuances that should be mentioned here.

Naming of Tests. First, we've covered a test called the independent-samples, pooled-variance t test. This is a very commonly used test. It's used whenever we wish to test whether there is a group difference in the mean of a quantitative variable.

The reader should understand, though, that there are many different "*t*" tests. Tests are named after the sampling distribution of the test statistic. So in addition to the *t* test we covered here, there is a *t* test for a correlation coefficient, a *t* test for a regression coefficient, a *t* test for a difference in means of dependent samples, and so forth. The reader should not be confused by this.

Statistical vs. Clinical Significance. When we declare that the result of a test of hypothesis is "statistically significant," all we're saying is we believe that H_0 is false. We're not saying *how* false it is, however. With a large enough sample size, virtually any test of hypothesis will be statistically significant. We must then ask ourselves whether the test results appear to be *clinically significant*. With a large enough sample in the diet study, for example, we might find that a difference of 0.03 in mean PSA between diet groups is statistically significant. But it would not be considered of any real clinical consequence. This is one reason why confidence intervals are useful. With them, we have a good idea what the true parameter value is. Then the subject-matter specialist can make a determination of whether or not it represents a clinically significant finding.

De-emphasis on Formulas. So far in this primer we have only considered the formulas for two test statistics for testing hypotheses: the large-sample test about a population mean—also called a *z* test—and the independent-samples, pooled-variance *t* test. In both cases, the reader has hopefully seen how the test statistic is measuring the discrepancy between what's actually observed in the sample, and what you'd expect to observe if H_0 were true. Once you understand what a test statistic is measuring, it's not necessary for us to examine the construction of every one. Rather, you know that the larger the test statistic value, the more discrepant sample results are from what H_0 would predict. The crux of the test is the *p* value, of course. And we have seen how to interpret those.

P *Values, Revisited*

Nevertheless, because the *p* value plays such a huge role in statistics, let's take another look at it in this final section. Once again, we turn to the GSS, but this time we use several years of GSS data. What we do is to consider two variables and examine whether there is a gender difference in the means of each. The first variable is labeled "SATJOB" and is described below (Table 4.2). The second variable is labeled "JOBINC" and its description follows the first (Table 4.3).

The sample sizes for the two variables are 38,292 for SATJOB and 19,625 for JOBINC. Now, let's pretend these are actually the populations answering these questions instead of just large samples. What we will do is to randomly sample from these "populations" and then conduct tests to see if there is a gender difference in each variable.

Table 4.2 Distribution of job satisfaction for GSS respondents

SATJOB	JOB OR HOUSEWORK

Description of the Variable
181. On the whole, how satisfied are you with the work you do?

Percent	N	Value	Label
47.6	18,239	1	VERY SATISFIED
38.2	14,632	2	MOD. SATISFIED
10.0	3,818	3	A LITTLE DISSAT
4.2	1,603	4	VERY DISSATISFIED
	13,254	0	IAP
	143	8	DK
	1,354	9	NA
100.0	53,043		Total

Properties	
Data type:	numeric
Missing-data codes:	0,8,9
Mean:	1.71
Std Dev:	.81
Record/column:	1/687

Selected Study: GSS 1972-2008 Cumulative Dataset

Table 4.3 Distribution of importance of high income from a job for GSS respondents

JOBINC	HIGH INCOME

Description of the Variable
183a. Would you please look at this card and tell me which one thing on this list you would most prefer in a job? b. Which comes next? c. Which is third most important? d. Which is fourth most important? HIGH INCOME

Percent	N	Value	Label
21.3	4,173	1	MOST IMPT
24.9	4,893	2	SECOND
30.4	5,971	3	THIRD
17.8	3,492	4	FOURTH
5.6	1,096	5	FIFTH
	32,812	0	IAP
	606	9	NA
100.0	53,043		Total

Properties	
Data type:	numeric
Missing-data codes:	0,8,9
Mean:	2.62
Std Dev:	1.16
Record/column:	1/689

Table 4.4 Mean job satisfaction scores for males and females in the GSS

Selected Study: GSS 1972-2008 Cumulative Dataset

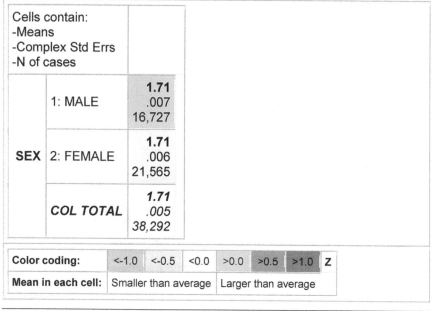

SDA 3.4: Means
GSS 1972-2008 Cumulative Dataset
Apr 21, 2010 (Wed 10:14 AM PDT)

Variables					
Role	**Name**	**Label**	**Range**	**MD**	**Dataset**
Dependent	**SATJOB**	JOB OR HOUSEWORK	1-4	0,8,9	1
Row	**SEX**	RESPONDENTS SEX	1-2	0	1

Main Statistics

Cells contain:
-Means
-Complex Std Errs
-N of cases

	1: MALE	**1.71** .007 16,727
SEX	2: FEMALE	**1.71** .006 21,565
	COL TOTAL	**1.71** .005 38,292

Color coding:	<-1.0	<-0.5	<0.0	>0.0	>0.5	>1.0	Z
Mean in each cell:	Smaller than average			Larger than average			

There is *absolutely no gender difference* on SATJOB in the "population," as we see here, since the means for males and females are exactly the same—1.71 (Table 4.4).

But there *is* a gender difference on JOBINC in "the population," as the following shows (Table 4.5). The means are 2.57 for males and 2.65 for females. Thus, there's a slight tendency for women to rate high income as being of lesser importance in a job, compared to males.

Table 4.5 Mean importance of high income for males and females in the GSS

SDA 3.4: Means
GSS 1972-2008 Cumulative Dataset
Apr 21, 2010 (Wed 12:00 PM PDT)

Variables					
Role	Name	Label	Range	MD	Dataset
Dependent	**JOBINC**	HIGH INCOME	1-5	0,8,9	1
Row	**SEX**	RESPONDENTS SEX	1-2	0	1

Main Statistics

Cells contain: -Means -Complex Std Errs -N of cases		
	1: MALE	**2.57** .016 8,758
SEX	2: FEMALE	**2.65** .015 10,867
	COL TOTAL	**2.62** *.013* *19,625*

Color coding:	<-1.0	<-0.5	<0.0	>0.0	>0.5	>1.0	Z
Mean in each cell:	Smaller than average			Larger than average			

Sampling from "The Population"

What we did next was to take a 3 % random sample from each "population." And then we used the independent-samples, pooled-variance t test to test for mean differences in each variable by gender. Here are the results (Table 4.6), using a software program called SAS. The means for males and females, respectively, on each

Table 4.6 SAS output showing *T* tests for gender differences in job satisfaction and the importance of high income

```
                        The TTEST Procedure

                           Statistics

                 Lower CL          Upper CL  Lower CL          Upper CL
Variable  sex       N    Mean    MEAN    Mean   Std Dev  Std Dev  Std Dev  Std Err

satjob    males     489  1.6751  1.7464  1.8178  0.7555   0.8029   0.8566   0.0363
          1
satjob    females   657  1.6329  1.6971  1.7613  0.7951   0.838    0.886    0.0327
          2
satjob    Diff (1-2)     -0.047  0.0493  0.1458  0.7908   0.8232   0.8584   0.0492


jobinc    males     253  2.3838  2.5257  2.6676  1.0543   1.1462   1.2559   0.0721
          1
jobinc    females   327  2.6789  2.8012  2.9235  1.0442   1.1243   1.2178   0.0622
          2
jobinc    Diff (1-2)     -0.462  -0.276  -0.089  1.0721   1.1339   1.2033   0.0949


                             T-Tests

        Variable    Method         Variances    DF     t Value   Pr > |t|

        satjob      Pooled         Equal        1144    1.00      0.3161
        satjob      Satterthwaite  Unequal      1075    1.01      0.3131
        jobinc      Pooled         Equal        578     -2.90     0.0038
        jobinc      Satterthwaite  Unequal      537     -2.89     0.0039


                       Equality of Variances

        Variable    Method     Num DF   Den DF   F Value   Pr > F

        satjob      Folded F    656      488      1.09     0.3135
        jobinc      Folded F    252      326      1.04     0.7409
```

variable, are in the column that is **in bold and underlined**, Males are group 1, and females are group 2. (Right after that are the *t* test results for whether mean differences by gender are significant.) As you can see, the *sample* means for both variables differ by gender. This is the result of sampling variability in the case of SATJOB, since, as we saw above, the population means are *identical*.

What do the *t* tests have to tell us about whether these mean differences are significant? Below the means, under "*T*-Tests" we have bolded and underlined the *t* test results (the other *t* test does not assume equal population variances; no matter—it gives the same results as the *t* test we've studied). As you can see, the *p* value for the SATJOB test is not significant; $p = 0.3161$. But the *p* value for the JOBINC test *is* significant; $p = 0.0038$. So in both cases, the *p* values are telling us what the correct decision should be: don't reject the null hypothesis that there's no gender difference on SATJOB, but *do* reject the null hypothesis that there's no gender difference in JOBINC. And from the sample results for the latter, we'd conclude that women are lower on the importance of income in a job. As we've seen, this would be correct. As a final comment: another way to interpret the *p* value is that it's the *probability the sample results only apply to your particular sample and not to the larger population from which your sample was drawn.*

Application: *T* Tests and Statistical Power in Action

Gender Difference in Physician Salaries

Jagsi et al. (2012) were interested in exploring potential gender inequity in physician salaries. Of interest was whether gender disparities in pay could be explained by specialization, work hours, productivity, and other job choices made by men and women, as opposed to discrimination based purely on gender. Their sample consisted of 800 physicians awarded National Institutes of Health career development awards in 2000–2003 and who continued to work at academic institutions. In Tables 1 and 2 of the article, they report associations between gender and various characteristics. They show average annual salaries for females and males of $167,669 and $200,433, respectively, with a mean difference of $32,764 favoring the males. Is this a significant difference? The *t* test for a difference produced a *p* value reported as "<0.001." Therefore, this mean salary difference between men and women physicians was quite significant. On the other hand, this is a salary gap that is not adjusted for other factors—work hours, productivity, etc.—that might account for the gender difference. We will see in Chap. 6 how these other factors can be adjusted for when we study multiple regression. In the meantime, we could consider whether there are gender differences on some of these other factors. Jagsi et al. use a *t* test to show that there is a significant difference in the average number of publications according to gender, with women's mean number of publications being 26.7 and men's mean being 33.3 ($p < 0.001$). Similarly, there is a significant gender difference in average weekly work hours, with women's and men's means being 58.1 and 63.2, respectively ($p < 0.001$). These findings suggest that, on average, men have more publications and put in more work hours than women do. In Chap. 6 we will consider to what extent these types of characteristics accounted for the gender gap in salary in their study.

Power Considerations in Hydroxychloroquine Study

In the aforementioned Paton and associates (2012) study of hydroxychloroquine vs. placebo in slowing the progression of HIV disease, the primary endpoint was (p. 356) "the change from baseline to week 48 in activation of CD8 cells, as shown by percentage of cells expressing CD38+ and HLA-DR+." The researchers invoke power considerations to explain their choice of sample size (p. 356):

> The sample size was estimated for the primary endpoint as follows. We proposed that a reduction in CD8 cell activation from 46 % to 35 % (ie, a 25 % reduction) would be a realistic goal of hydroxychloroquine therapy given the magnitude of the changes usually seen with antiretroviral therapy. Models indicate that this level of reduction would be expected to decrease the relative hazard for disease progression by at least 50 %. The standard deviation for the reduction was estimated as 15 %. With a 2-sided α of .05 and a power of 90 %, a total of 80 patients would be required.

We see first that the estimate of a power value of 0.90 (reported as a percent) required an estimate of how much of an effect hydroxychloroquine would have, compared to placebo, in reducing CD8 cell activation. Under the null hypothesis of no effect of treatment, we would expect no reduction in CD8 cell activation, compared to placebo. So a 25 % reduction is posed as the effect of hydroxychloroquine that they would like to be able to detect with probability 0.90. Second, the standard deviation of the primary endpoint plays a role in power calculation and so also required an estimate (15 %). And third, the alpha-level (α) also needed to be specified, along with whether the test would be one- or two tailed ("-sided").

Power in the Arterial Inflammation Study

Subramanian et al. (2012) hypothesized that arterial wall inflammation is increased in HIV patients, compared to those not infected with HIV having similar cardiac risk factors. To test this hypothesis, they performed two separate comparisons. One compared 27 HIV patients without cardiac disease with 27 non-HIV control participants without atherosclerotic disease and matched to the HIV group on age, sex, and Framingham risk score. The other comparison was of the aforementioned 27 HIV patients with 54 non-HIV controls with known atherosclerotic disease who were matched to the HIV group by sex. The researchers describe the primary endpoint thus (p. 380): "The ascending aorta was chosen for measurement. The target-to-background ratio (TBR) was calculated by dividing the mean arterial standardized uptake value (SUV) by the mean venous SUV." They describe their power calculations as follows (p. 381): "With 54 patients in each 2-group comparison, the study was powered at 85 % with a 2-sided significance level of 0.05, to detect a 0.83-SD difference between the groups." Here, again, the group difference that they would like to be able to detect is stated explicitly: a 0.83-standard deviation (SD) difference in the TBR between HIV and control group in each comparison.

Next. At this point, we have covered several basic topics in statistics. This includes causality and causal inferences, descriptive uses of statistics, and the logic of inferential techniques such as confidence intervals and the test of hypothesis. A particularly useful test, the independent-samples pooled-variance *t* test has been discussed. This test is useful whenever we have a binary treatment and a quantitative study endpoint. However, there are many other scenarios involving treatment and response that remain to be covered. These include having a treatment with more than two levels and either a quantitative or qualitative response, as well as having a quantitative "treatment" and a quantitative response, or having a quantitative treatment and a qualitative response. How all these situations are handled is the subject of the next chapter.

Chapter 5
Bivariate Statistical Techniques

In the preceding chapters we covered fundamental definitions, concepts, and tests in statistics. In this chapter, we will go beyond the basics to explore more advanced statistical tools. We begin by revisiting the steak-diet data and discussing a nonparametric alternative to the *independent-samples, pooled-variance t test* that we covered earlier. We then segue to other types of analyses for comparing groups on a study endpoint. These techniques vary according to how both "group" and study endpoint are measured. We will also see these statistics "in action" by looking at examples taken from the medical literature.

A Nonparametric Test for the Steak-Diet Example

Recall the steak diet, PSA example from the previous chapter. There we tested whether a steak diet results in an elevated PSA level, compared to a balanced diet. We used a parametric test, the independent-samples *t* test for this purpose. And we failed to reject the null hypothesis. The *t* test rests on several assumptions about the data that we did not really investigate. Nevertheless, the *t* test is robust to violations of its assumptions provided that the sample sizes in each group are the same, and both are over about 30. However, the diet study only had six men in each group—far short of the recommended sample size. Therefore, perhaps we should retest the research hypothesis using an approach that doesn't rest on so many assumptions. An ideal candidate is the *Wilcoxon Rank Sum Test* (*WRST*), a nonparametric test (Ott 1988). Nonparametric tests, including the WRST, make no assumptions about how the study endpoint is distributed in the respective subpopulations under study (e.g., men on a balanced vs. a steak diet). The only assumptions for the WRST are that the endpoint is a quantitative variable and that the samples are independent. This contrasts with the *t* test, which additionally assumes that PSA is normally distributed in each subpopulation and that the variance of PSA is also the same for each subpopulation.

A. DeMaris and S.H. Selman, *Converting Data into Evidence: A Statistics Primer for the Medical Practitioner*, DOI 10.1007/978-1-4614-7792-1_5,
© Springer Science+Business Media New York 2013

Computing the WRST

The hypotheses for the WRST are simple:

Null hypothesis: the two subpopulations are identical.
Research hypothesis: subpopulation 2 (steak-diet group) is shifted to the right of subpopulation 1 (balanced-diet group).

As is evident here, the WRST doesn't compare means. Rather, it simply considers whether the collection of study endpoints for each subpopulation is the same. If one collection of endpoints tends to be greater than the other, then we say that it is "shifted to the right" of the other. This is what we expect, since we anticipate that the collection of PSA values for the steak-diet subpopulation will tend to be greater than those for the control subpopulation. The way this is tested is as follows. We combine the PSA values from both groups into one sample. We then rank all of these values from lowest (1) to highest (12). If there were tied values, they would be assigned the same rank. That common rank would be the average of the ranks the tied values would have gotten had they been different. So if the fifth and sixth ranked values were the same, they would both get the rank 5.5. The next rank assigned would be 7, and so forth. Here are the control and steak-diet groups' PSA values again (Table 5.1), with ranks assigned (in parentheses):

The test statistic is simply the sum of the ranks for group 2, the steak-diet group. That sum is 42. Now, if the subpopulations have identical endpoint values, then the sum of the ranks should be about the same for each group. If the rank sum for one of the groups is unusually large, this is evidence that the subpopulations are not the same. Under the research hypothesis, we would expect the sum of ranks for the steak group to be large. It turns out to be 42. Is this large enough to reject the null? For this purpose we have to look the sum up in a special table for the Wilcoxon test (such as Table 3 in the Appendix of Ott 1988). It turns out that, given a sample size of 6 in each group, we would need the sum of ranks in the group with higher values to be at least 52 to reject the null. (The table automatically adjusts the critical value needed for rejection of the null when the samples are of different sizes.) So, consistent with what we found using the t test, we fail again to reject the null hypothesis here. And once again we conclude there's not enough evidence to say that PSA levels are elevated by a steak diet.

Table 5.1 Control (balanced-diet) and steak-diet groups with values rank-ordered from lowest to highest

Control		Steak	
2.3	(2)	2.0	(1)
2.7	(4)	2.6	(3)
3.0	(5)	3.1	(6)
4.0	(7)	4.9	(9)
4.6	(8)	7.0	(11)
6.0	(10)	7.5	(12)

Bivariate Statistics

To this point, we have used both the t test and the WRST to compare two groups on a quantitative study endpoint. Both tests are examples of *bivariate* statistical techniques. "Bivariate" refers to the fact that there are two variables involved: treatment and response. (Sometimes, however, analysts will call this "univariate" analysis because there is only one explanatory variable—treatment—involved; nevertheless "bivariate" is the correct statistical term.) The treatment in all cases so far has been two-valued: steak diet vs. control diet or men vs. women (in the GSS data). The treatment in a study is also called the *independent variable*, the *predictor*, the *covariate*, or the *regressor*, depending on the type of analysis used. The response variable in the diet study was the PSA level. The response variable in the GSS was physician stewardship. Both are quantitative variables. In the diet study, we examined whether there was a difference in mean PSA between the groups. Another way to say this is that we examined whether there was an *association* (or relationship) between diet and PSA level. In the following sections, armed with the terminology and rationale behind hypothesis tests, we will look at a variety of bivariate procedures designed to tell us whether an association exists between two variables. The type of test used depends on the level of measurement of the two variables. We've examined the case in which we have a quantitative response and a binary, qualitative treatment. There are many other scenarios to consider. Showing association is typically the first step in marshaling evidence for causality. With random assignment to treatment groups, it is often the only step we need. But with nonexperimental studies there is much more to be done. We will illustrate this latter principle when we discuss regression modeling and statistical control in Chap. 6.

Bivariate Analysis: Other Scenarios

Continuing with bivariate tests, we consider other scenarios. For example, we might have a quantitative response and a qualitative treatment with more than two categories. Or we might have a qualitative response and a qualitative treatment. Or, lastly, we could have a quantitative response and a quantitative treatment. We will cover each of these situations in turn. In that we know the rationale behind, and general interpretation of, a test statistic, we won't always give the calculations for test statistics from here on out. In some instances, we'll simply identify the name of the appropriate test statistic. Also, it should be noted that there are three aspects to consider in examining bivariate association. First, we wish to know whether the association *exists* in the study population, not just in our particular sample. This is the purpose of the test of hypothesis and associated test statistic and p value. The null hypothesis typically posits that there is no association. So if we reject it, we conclude there is an association in the population. Second, if there is an association, we wish to know its *direction*. This refers to the nature of the association, or how the treatment affects the response. Third, if there is an association, we wish to know how *strong* it is. The strength of association refers to how well knowing the treatment that was applied allows us to predict the value of the response. In the diet study above, had the association been significant (i.e., we rejected the null and accepted the alternative hypothesis), the direction would have been stated as "a meat diet results in a *higher* average PSA level, compared to a balanced diet," since that is what the sample results suggested. The strength of association when examining the association between a qualitative dichotomous treatment and a quantitative response is denoted by r^2 and its formula is

$$r^2 = \frac{t^2}{t^2 + \mathrm{df}},$$

where df is the degrees of freedom of the t statistic. In the diet example, we have

$$r^2 = \frac{0.68^2}{0.68^2 + 10} = 0.044.$$

Measures of strength of association usually range in absolute value between 0 and 1.0. Zero represents no association whatsoever and 1.0 represents perfect association—the response is perfectly determined by the treatment. In this case, a value of 0.044 represents a pretty weak association. We shall have more to say about r^2 below.

Qualitative Treatment with More Than Two Levels: ANOVA

Recall that the diet study actually had three treatment levels, consisting of control, steak, and vegetarian diets, as shown in Table 2.1. Let's reconsider the results of the study using all three conditions. You might think we could just do three different t tests to test the differences between the three pairs of means that result from the groups. However, if we do that, we begin to accumulate the probability of a Type I error across multiple tests. This means that the chance of making at least one Type I error when we do, say, three tests, is greater than if we just do one test. In fact, that chance is 0.143 if we do three tests. If we were to do ten tests, which is what we'd be doing if there were five treatment groups under study, the probability of making at least one Type I error increases to 0.401. The phenomenon of an elevated probability of rejecting true null hypotheses merely because you're doing multiple tests is called *capitalization on chance*. To avoid that, we do one test for whether there is any difference between the three group means in the population, with a Type I error rate of 0.05. The hypotheses are:

Null hypothesis: there is no difference in mean PSA among the three treatment groups.
Research hypothesis: at least one mean PSA is different than the others.

Table 5.2 Crosstabulation of erectile function with treatment assignment

Erectile function	Treatment assignment		
	PDE5 + ASA	PDE5	Total
Erection	18	6	24
	(72 %)	(32 %)	(55 %)
Flaccid	7	13	20
	(28 %)	(68 %)	(45 %)
Total	25	19	44

The analytic procedure we're using is called analysis of variance or ANOVA for short. It's an extension of the t test we showed above. (In fact, the t test is the specialized case of an ANOVA with just two groups.) The test statistic here is the F test. (With just two groups, F and t are closely related; in fact, $t = \sqrt{F}$.) In the diet study, the three group means are 3.77 (balanced diet), 4.52 (meat diet), and 2.88 (vegetarian diet). Although it looks like the means are different, based on the sample, the F test statistic is only 1.32 here, with a p value of 0.296. So the results are nonsignificant and we cannot reject the null hypothesis. Were we able to reject the null, the next question would be which pairs of means are different? That is, which means are different from which others, considered one pair at a time? When each pair of means is tested to see if the difference is significant following a significant F test, these subsequent tests are referred to as *post hoc* tests. They would be addressed using a *multiple-comparison procedure*, such as the Tukey, Bonferroni, or Scheffe procedures. All of these techniques allow us to do multiple comparisons of pairs of means to see which are significantly different, while holding the overall Type I error rate across all comparisons to 0.05. In this case, however, we needn't bother, since the F test was insignificant. For ANOVA, the direction of association is specified by talking about which means are larger or smaller than others. And the strength of association is again measured using an r^2, with a different formula, in this case. For the diet study, the r^2 for the ANOVA is 0.15, again on a scale from 0 to 1. Although it's larger than the 0.044 with just two groups, we shouldn't make much of this since (a) the association is not significant, and (b) r^2 is artificially inflated in value when you have more treatment levels and the n is small, as in this case.

Qualitative Treatment and Qualitative Response: χ^2

When both treatment and response are qualitative, we use the *chi-squared* test statistic, denoted χ^2, to test the null hypothesis of no association. (A related statistic, *Fisher's exact test*, is used with very small samples; however, we will not cover this technique in this primer.) As an example, suppose we're interested in determining whether aspirin use can improve erectile function when used in conjunction with a PDE5 inhibitor. For our study, we randomly assign men to be treated with PDE5 and ASA ($n_1 = 25$) or to be treated with PDE5 alone ($n_2 = 19$). The results of the study are shown in Table 5.2.

This type of table is referred to as a *crosstabulation* or *contingency* table. The "total" column in the right margin of the table shows the *unconditional distribution* of erectile function for the sample as a whole. Thus, 24 men, or 55 %, have erections and 20 men, or 45 %, are flaccid. Each column inside the table shows the distribution of erectile function conditional on being in a particular treatment group, and therefore these are referred to as the *conditional distributions* on erectile function, given treatment group. The sample data show an association between the variables whenever the conditional distributions on the response are different from its unconditional distribution. That is the case here, since fully 72 % of men in the PDE5 + ASA group have erections, compared with only 32 % in the PDE5 group. If there were no association, you would expect both conditional distributions to be identical to the unconditional distribution. That is, there would be a 55–45 % distribution on erectile function in each treatment group, with 55 % of each treatment group having experienced erections. That would indicate that the percent having erections was unrelated to treatment group. However, there does appear to be an association here. Is this association significant? That is, can we reject the null hypothesis of no association between these variables in the "population"? The assumptions for the chi-squared test are: first, that we have a random sample from the population, and second, that the sample is "large enough." There are standard rules in statistics textbooks regarding necessary sample size, but these are a bit too restrictive. A better rule of thumb is that average cell size should be at least 5 (Agresti 1990). In this case the total n is 44 and there are four cells, giving us an average cell size of $44/4 = 11$, which is adequate. The hypotheses can be stated:

Null hypothesis: there is no association between treatment and response.
Research hypothesis: there is an association between treatment and response.

The test statistic, as mentioned, is χ^2, and like the t test it has an associated df, which, in this case is 1. Its value for these data is 7.13, with a p value of 0.008. This is significant, so we would reject the null and conclude that PDE5 + ASA leads to a higher likelihood of an erection, compared to PDE5 alone. (Notice the directional conclusion, even though the research hypothesis was nondirectional or two tailed.) On the one hand, this is sufficient for our purposes. On the other hand, as the χ^2 statistic is easy to calculate and as its calculation is instructive for illustrating the rationale behind a test statistic, let's delve a little further.

Calculating the χ^2 Value

Recall that a test statistic measures the discrepancy between what is observed in the sample and what you'd expect to observe under the null. To show how the χ^2 statistic illustrates this principle, let's calculate the χ^2 for this table. What we *observe* are the cell counts in the table, that is, the numbers 18, 6, 7, and 13. What we need to know is what we would *expect* to observe if the null hypothesis were true. If there were no relationship between these two variables, then the conditional distributions—the

Table 5.3 Crosstabulation of erectile function with treatment assignment under perfect association

Erectile function	Treatment assignment		Total
	PDE5 + ASA	PDE5	
Erection	25	0	25
	(100 %)	(0 %)	(57 %)
Flaccid	0	19	19
	(0 %)	(100 %)	(43 %)
Total	25	19	44

proportions erect vs. flaccid given treatment group—would be identical with the 55–45 % breakdown observed in the unconditional distribution of Erectile Function. That means that we would expect to see 55 % of the 25 men, or 13.75 men (the expected count is left in decimal form even though 0.75 % of a man is nonsensical!), in the PDE5 + ASA group with erections and 45 %, or 11.25, of them flaccid. Similarly, we'd expect to see 55 % of the 19 men, or 10.45 men, in the PDE5 group with erections and 45 % of them, or 8.55 of them, flaccid. The numbers 13.75, 11.25, 10.45, and 8.55 are then the corresponding numbers we would expect to see in the cells of the table if the null hypothesis were true. To measure how large of a discrepancy this represents, compared to what we actually observe, the χ^2 statistic is calculated as

$$\chi^2 = \frac{(18-13.75)^2}{13.75} + \frac{(6-10.45)^2}{10.45} + \frac{(7-11.25)^2}{11.25} + \frac{(13-8.55)^2}{8.55} = 7.13.$$

Hence, we see that χ^2 is tapping the discrepancy between observed and expected (under the null) cell counts in each cell. The reason for squaring the difference between the observed and expected cell count in each case is that the observed–expected differences are both positive and negative over all the cells. So they would tend to cancel each other out in a straight sum.

Minimum and Maximum Values of χ^2

If all of the observed cell counts were exactly equal to the expected cell counts, χ^2 would equal zero, correctly indicating no discrepancy between observed and expected cell counts. This would imply that there is no association between the two variables, whatsoever. On the other hand, with the most extreme departure of observed from expected cell counts possible, χ^2 would equal n, the table total. This would indicate a perfect association in which each conditional distribution would show a 100–0 % split, except in opposite directions. Table 5.3 demonstrates what the erectile function data would look like if the association between treatment and erectile function were "perfect":

Here we note that all of the PDE5 + ASA group have erections and all of the PDE5 group are flaccid. So erection status is perfectly predictable knowing treatment group. Or we could say that erection status is perfectly determined by

treatment-group status, without error. One almost never encounters perfect association in real data, however. At any rate, at this point it should be clear how χ^2 is tapping the observed vs. expected cell count discrepancy via the way it is calculated.
Letting O = observed cell count and E = expected cell count, the general formula for
the χ^2 statistic is

$$\sum_{\text{cells}} \frac{(O-E)^2}{E},$$

where the "Σ" symbol means to sum over the cells of the table the expression that
appears to the right of it.

Measuring the Strength of Association

Finally, how strong is the association in Table 5.2? There is a measure for this that
is equivalent to r^2. It's denoted Φ^2 (phi-squared) and is computed as χ^2/n, which, in
this case, equals $7.13/44 = 0.16$. The association is weak to moderate in strength. As
the χ^2 value can range from 0 to n, the Φ^2 value can range from 0 to 1.0. Another
measure of strength of association that is particularly interpretable is the odds ratio
(Agresti and Finlay 2009). In Table 5.2, the probability of an erection for the
PDE5 + ASA group is 0.72. The *odds* of an erection for this group is the ratio of this
probability to the probability of being flaccid: Odds = 0.72/0.28 = 2.57. (Although it
may seem grammatically incorrect, the odds is treated as singular.) That is, the probability of having an erection is over two-and-a-half times as great as the probability
of remaining flaccid. For the PDE5 group, on the other hand, the probability of an
erection is 0.32, which means the odds of an erection is 0.32/0.68 = 0.47. So the odds
of an erection is much greater in the PDE5 + ASA group. To quantify this difference,
we can compute the ratio of the two odds: *Odds Ratio (OR)* = 2.57/0.47 = 5.47. This
is telling us that the odds of an erection for the PDE5 + ASA group is 5.47 times
greater than the odds for the PDE5 group. The odds ratio is an alternative measure
of the strength of association between two variables. Its drawback in this regard,
however, is that it is not bounded by 0 and 1. Therefore, it's harder to get a sense of
how strong the relationship is, especially considering that the odds ratio can range
from 0 to infinity. The odds ratio, however, is ideal for expressing the size of the
"effect" that one variable has on the other in the technique called "logistic regression" that will be covered in Chap. 7. Another measure of strength that is related to
the odds ratio is the *relative risk* (RR). The relative risk is the ratio of probabilities,
rather than odds. So the relative risk of an erection for the PDE5 + ASA group, vs.
the PDE5 group is 0.72/0.32 = 2.25. We would say that an erection is 2.25 times
more likely for the PDE5 + ASA group than it is for the PDE5 group. Notice that the
RR is not the same as the OR here. And this is usually the case, unless the probability
in both groups is very small, say 0.05 or less. In that case, RR and OR are virtually
the same.

Table 5.4 BMI, PSA, and MIN for a sample of five men

BMI (x)	PSA (y)	MIN	$(BMI - \bar{x})$	$(PSA - \bar{y})$	Crossproduct: $(BMI - \bar{x})(PSA - \bar{y})$
22	2.5	13	−3.8	−0.06	0.228
24	1.5	15	−1.8	−1.06	1.908
25	2.6	14	−0.8	0.04	−0.032
28	2.4	12	2.2	−0.16	−0.352
30	3.8	12	4.2	1.24	5.208

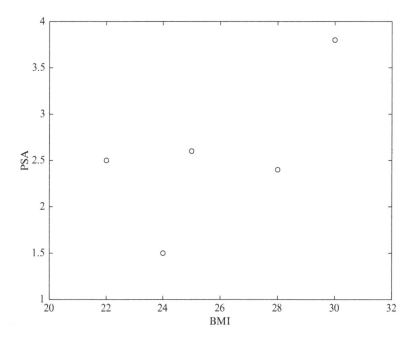

Fig. 5.1 Scatterplot of PSA (*vertical axis*) against BMI (*horizontal axis*)

Quantitative Treatment and Response: The Correlation Coefficient

Finally we come to the situation in which both treatment and response are quantitative. For example, the first three columns of Table 5.4 present data for five men on their BMI (body mass index), their PSA, and MIN (the number of minutes they can run on a treadmill before their heart rate reaches 125).

Suppose that our research hypotheses are that PSA increases with BMI but falls with MIN. That is, we think that being overweight, as indexed by a higher BMI, is associated with elevated PSA levels. But we think that keeping fit, as indexed by a higher MIN, is associated with lower PSA levels. First, in Fig. 5.1, let's examine a scatterplot of PSA against BMI:

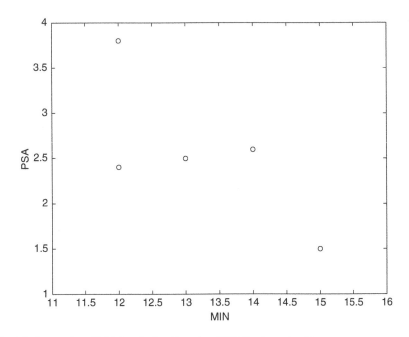

Fig. 5.2 Scatterplot of PSA (*vertical axis*) against MIN (*horizontal axis*)

A scatterplot shows each man's pair of BMI and PSA values as a "point" (symbolized by "o") on a plot. The horizontal axis tabulates BMI values and the vertical axis tabulates PSA values. Any given point shows the intersection of a given man's BMI score with his PSA score. For example, the first point on the left is for a man with a BMI of 22 (as seen by drawing a line from the point straight down to where it intersects the BMI axis) and a PSA of 2.5 (as seen by drawing a line parallel to the BMI axis until it intersects the PSA axis). The second point, moving right, is for a man with a BMI of 24 and a PSA of 1.5 and so forth. The pattern of points conveys the nature of the association between BMI and PSA. In that the points tend to move upward as we go up in BMI, it appears that higher BMI values are associated with higher PSA values. Similarly, Fig. 5.2 shows a scatterplot of PSA against MIN:

In this case, the points are moving downward as we go up in MIN, indicating that longer endurance on the treadmill is associated with lower PSA values. At this juncture, the data are consistent with our hypotheses. But we need to subject that hypothesis to a formal test. To do that, we need a statistical measure of the association between PSA and each other factor. The *Pearson Product–Moment Correlation Coefficient*, or Correlation Coefficient for short, denoted by r, is designed to capture the association between two quantitative variables. It tells us how one variable "behaves" as the other increases in value. There are four options. It can increase. It can decrease. It can alternate between increasing and decreasing. Or it can fluctuate randomly. The correlation coefficient can detect either of the first two options or the last option well. It is particularly poor at detecting the third option (see below for an example). For the time being, however, let us regard the association between BMI and PSA.

Since we think that BMI has a causal impact on PSA level, let us denote BMI as x and PSA as y. (It is conventional to label cause and effect as x and y, respectively.) To compute the correlation coefficient, first we will calculate the *covariance* between x and y, denoted cov(x, y). This is done as follows. We create deviation scores for each x and y value, denoted ($x - \bar{x}$) and ($y - \bar{y}$) for x and y, respectively. For each variable, deviation scores are computed by subtracting the variable's mean from each of its values. We then multiply these deviation scores together for each unit. The result is called the *crossproduct*. We then sum these crossproducts up and divide that sum by $n - 1$. This gives us the sample covariance. In statistical parlance, the formula is

$$\mathrm{cov}(x, y) = \frac{\sum (x - \bar{x})(y - \bar{y})}{n - 1},$$

where "Σ," once again, indicates summing—in this instance, it is the crossproducts that are summed over all the cases.

The key calculations for the correlation between BMI and PSA are shown in columns 4, 5, and 6 of Table 5.4. The mean of BMI is 25.8 and the mean of PSA is 2.56. The sum of the crossproducts for the five men is 6.96, hence cov(x, y) is 6.96/ $(5 - 1) = 1.74$. That this is positive means that the variables are increasing together. That is, higher values of BMI are associated with higher values of PSA, and lower values of BMI are associated with lower PSAs. (This is fairly evident in the table.) Although this is good information, cov(x, y) isn't very useful as a descriptive measure of association because its size depends on the units of measurement. Thus, there is no way of judging whether a covariance of 1.74 is a strong association or a weak association. For this reason, we "standardize" the covariance by dividing it by the product of the respective standard deviations of x and y (denoted, respectively, s_x and s_y). By mathematical theorem, cov(x, y) cannot exceed, in absolute value, the product of s_x with s_y. The resulting measure is the correlation coefficient, and its range is from −1.0 to +1.0. Its formula is

$$r = \frac{\mathrm{cov}(x, y)}{s_x s_y}.$$

The standard deviations are 3.19 for BMI and 0.82 for PSA. Thus, r here is 1.74/ $[(3.19)(0.82)] = 0.67$. This represents a fairly strong positive association. On the other hand, the correlation between MIN and PSA is −0.74 (these calculations are not shown in the table), which represents a fairly strong negative association. So, at least in the sample, our hunches appear to be supported: an increasing BMI is associated with an increasing PSA but an increasing MIN is associated with a decreasing PSA. If a correlation is approximately zero, it can mean one of two things. First, it can mean that y is fluctuating randomly as x increases, showing no identifiable pattern. This means there is no association between x and y. But a zero correlation can also mask a pattern of association between x and y that is *not linear*. Correlation is designed to detect only *linear* association and will miss nonlinear relationships. Finally, if r is −1.0 or +1.0, it means that y is perfectly determined by x. This is almost never observed with real data.

One somewhat artificial example of perfect determination, however, is the relationship between temperature in centigrade and temperature in Fahrenheit. For these two temperature measures, the correlation is 1.0. Why? Well, the formula for temperature in centigrade (C) as a function of temperature in Fahrenheit (F) is $C = -17.78 + 0.56F$. This formula shows that C is a *linear function of* (or formula involving) F. Technically, a linear formula (or function) is a weighted sum, i.e., it's the sum of variables (e.g., F) multiplied by constants (e.g., 0.56) added to potentially other constants (e.g., −17.78). If that formula perfectly determines y, as it does in the case of these two temperature measures, then the correlation is 1 in absolute value. But what happens if the formula involving x perfectly determines y but is not linear? For example, suppose our x values are −2, −1, 0, 1, 2, and the corresponding y values are 4, 1, 0, 1, 4. The correlation between x and y is zero in this case (as is easily verified). However, x perfectly determines y via the formula $y = x^2$. Nevertheless, as this is not a linear formula (since x is raised to a power rather than multiplied by a constant), r completely misses the association. The moral of this story is simple: if you suspect that x and y are related in a nonlinear fashion, don't rely on the correlation alone to test the association. (More about this when we get to regression modeling.)

Testing the Significance of R

Once we calculate the correlation coefficient, we want to test whether it is significant. That is, does a correlation exist in the target population? We denote the population correlation coefficient by ρ. Hence, our (two-tailed) hypotheses are as follows:

Null hypothesis: ρ is zero.
Research hypothesis: ρ is not zero.

The test statistic is a t statistic, again, calculated as

$$t = \frac{r}{\sqrt{\dfrac{1 - r^2}{n - 2}}}.$$

Table 5.5 PSA levels for
men in the diet-PSA study

Control	Steak
4.6	2.0
2.3	4.9
2.7	3.1
3.0	2.6
6.0	7.0
4.0	7.5

If the null hypothesis is true, this statistic has a t distribution with $n - 2$ df. For the BMI, PSA example, we have

$$t = \frac{0.67}{\sqrt{\frac{1 - 0.67^2}{5 - 2}}} = 1.56.$$

A t of 1.56 with $5 - 2 = 3$ df corresponds to a one-tailed p value of 0.11. So the correlation here is not significant. This isn't surprising, since the sample is too small to afford much power to detect a nonzero correlation in the population.

The Paired t Test: How Correlation Affects the Standard Error

Recall the t test for a difference of means that we performed in Chap. 4. When we have equal n in each group the formula was shown as

$$t = \frac{\bar{x}_2 - \bar{x}_1}{s_p \sqrt{\frac{2}{n}}}.$$

Let's write this formula slightly differently:

$$t = \frac{\bar{x}_2 - \bar{x}_1}{\sqrt{\frac{s_p^2}{n} + \frac{s_p^2}{n}}}. \tag{5.1}$$

These two formulas are exactly the same mathematically, but expressed differently. What's the point? The point is that there is another t test for a difference of means called the *paired t test*. But it is designed for the case in which the two sets of scores are for the *same cases*. Here are the diet data once again from Chap. 2, but just for the control (balanced-diet) and steak-diet conditions (Table 5.5):

Now suppose that instead of separate groups of men, these are the data for the *same six men*. First they are put on a balanced diet for 6 months, after which their

PSA levels are measured. Then they are put on a steak diet for the next 6 months, after which their PSA levels are measured again. Now the question is: is there a change in mean PSA from the control diet to the steak diet? In this case, we cannot any longer use the independent samples, pooled-variance t test to answer this question. Why? The reason is that the two sets of PSA scores are no longer independent. That is, they don't come from two unrelated groups of men; they're from the *same* men. So they are positively correlated. In fact, the correlation between the "control" and "steak" scores in Table 5.5 is 0.41. The two sets of scores are the product of *dependent sampling*: the data come as pairs of values "tied together" by virtue of some common source. In this case, the common source is the same man providing both sets of scores. In other cases, the common source is not as obvious. For example, if we had blood pressure data from husband and wife for several couples, each pair of blood pressure values for the same couple would be "tied together" by virtue of coming from the same couple. In that couples tend to be similar in their diet and their lifestyles, their blood pressure values are also probably positively correlated. Bottom line: to test for a mean difference between control and steak PSA values here, we have to take account of this positive correlation when calculating the standard error of the mean difference. That's the denominator of the t test statistic. Intuitively, if the scores in question are positively correlated, then their means, over repeated sampling, would also tend to be positively correlated. And this means that the mean differences over repeated sampling will tend to be smaller than they would be if the scores were from two unrelated groups of men. The formula for the paired t test is

$$t = \frac{\overline{x}_2 - \overline{x}_1}{\sqrt{\dfrac{s_1^2}{n} + \dfrac{s_2^2}{n} - \dfrac{2rs_1s_2}{n}}} \tag{5.2}$$

where s_1 and s_2 represent the standard deviations of the control and steak scores, respectively, and r represents the correlation between these two sets of scores. Compare this test to the one in (5.1). One difference, of course, is that in (5.2) the standard deviation of each group of scores is used in the denominator, rather than assuming that there is a common standard deviation (i.e., s_p) that applies to both sets of scores. But the more important difference is that the denominator of (5.2) has an extra term involving r that is being subtracted from the sum of the first two terms. This is adjusting for the dependence between the two sets of scores and results in a smaller denominator—which is the standard error of the mean difference in the numerator. This results in a test that is more likely to be significant for a given mean difference between the scores.

Recall that $s_1 = 1.38$ and $s_2 = 2.33$. Also, the means for the control and steak groups are 3.77 and 4.52, respectively. Thus, the paired t test statistic for these data turns out to be

$$t = \frac{4.52 - 3.77}{\sqrt{\dfrac{1.38^2}{6} + \dfrac{2.33^2}{6} - \dfrac{2(0.41)(1.38)(2.33)}{6}}} = 0.85.$$

Under the null hypothesis of no change in the mean PSA, this has a t distribution with 5 df. It's not significant. But notice that it is a larger t value than the t of 0.68 we found in Chap. 4 for the case in which these two sets of PSA values were assumed to be independent—from different men. That's because the standard error is smaller here: the denominator of the test statistic is 0.88, as opposed to 1.1, which was the denominator for the test in (5.1) that we found in the last chapter. Bottom line: the paired t test adjusts the standard error of the t test for the dependence between the two sets of scores in question. Because the scores virtually always show a positive correlation, this tends to reduce the standard error, compared to what it would be if the two sets of scores were independent. And this makes for a more sensitive test, i.e., one that is more likely to detect a significant difference. If the men were measured at more than just two times in the diet example, we'd employ an extension of the paired t test called *repeated-measures ANOVA*, which we will cover in the next chapter.

Summary of Bivariate Statistics

At this point, we've covered the bivariate statistical techniques necessary for testing hypotheses about an association between two variables under three scenarios: a qualitative treatment and a quantitative response, a qualitative treatment and a qualitative response, and a quantitative treatment and a quantitative response. However, we've left out one possibility: What should we do if we have a quantitative treatment and a qualitative response? In the bivariate context, it turns out that it makes no difference which variable is quantitative and which is qualitative. We use the same technique, either the two-sample t test, the paired t test, or ANOVA, depending on how many groups are represented by the qualitative variable. Thus, at this point, we've covered the major bivariate techniques you need to know. Periodically, you might encounter other bivariate statistics that were not covered here. These may include certain nonparametric procedures or procedures that are designed specifically for quantitative data representing only rank order on the attribute of interest. The latter include measures such as Spearman's rho, gamma, and Kendall's Tau B. In sum, even if one is not familiar with these particular statistics, the interpretation of test statistic, p value, direction of relationship, and strength of relationship are all by now familiar territory.

Application: Bivariate Statistics in Action

ANOVA: GGT and Alcohol Consumption

Tynjala and colleagues (2012) investigated the association between alcohol consumption and gamma-glutamyltransferase (GGT) enzyme in 18,889 respondents recruited via three independent cross-sectional surveys in Finland. Serum GGT activities are used as a biomarker of excessive alcohol consumption and liver dysfunction. There is currently substantial interest in serum GGT levels as a general indicator of health and disease (Tynjala et al. 2012). The survey involved physical measurements and laboratory tests, including the measurement of serum GGT. The authors classified respondents into four groups based on their pattern of alcohol consumption: abstainers, former drinkers, moderate drinkers, and heavy drinkers. They then examined how these groups differed in serum GGT using ANOVA, while controlling for potential confounding respondent characteristics. Here is how they report their analytic methodology (p. 559):

> Univariate differences between groups were determined with analysis of variance using the Bonferroni post hoc test for multiple comparisons. Logarithmic transformation of GGT data was used to obtain non-skewed distribution with homogeneity of variance. Age, BMI and the amount of smoked cigarettes per day were used as covariates in all analyses in order to avoid the effect of possible confounding factors. Values are expressed as mean ± SD. The statistical analyses were carried out using SPSS for Windows 19.0 (Chicago, IL, USA). A P-value of < 0.05 was considered statistically significant.

Let's "deconstruct" this description a bit. Notice the use of the term "univariate" in the first sentence. Technically, that is not correct. At the least, it is a bivariate analysis, with the independent variable being drinking status and the study endpoint being serum GGT. The Bonferroni post hoc test is essentially a t test for the mean difference in serum GGT between any two groups. But it corrects for capitalization on chance because with four groups, there are six total comparisons one can make between pairs of drinking-status groups. With the Bonferroni technique, the chance of making at least one Type I error in all six tests is kept at 0.05. They use the natural logarithm of serum GGT instead of raw serum GGT as the study endpoint to satisfy assumptions of ANOVA. These assumptions are that serum GGT is normally distributed in each drinking-status group and that the variance of GGT is the same in each group. When the original variable does not meet these assumptions, the logarithm of that variable typically does. The reference to age, BMI, and cigarettes smoked being used as "covariates" means that they are controlled in the analysis. In the next chapter we discuss the concept of statistical control. For the time being, let's just accept that, statistically, the four drinking groups are being "made the same" on these three factors in the ANOVA. The analyses were done with the statistical software package SPSS, and results were considered significant if p values were 0.05 or less. Their results are shown as figures, with men's and women's data analyzed separately (Fig. 5.3):

Here is how the authors describe these results in the narrative (p. 559):

> Among the subgroups, both men and women showed the lowest GGT values in abstainers (27.7 ± 1.6; 18.4 ± 1.7 U/l), the activities being significantly different from those observed in moderate drinkers (31.8 ± 1.8; 20.1 ± 1.7 U/l) (P < 0.001 for both) or heavy drinkers (56.9 ± 2.3; 30.8 ± 2.3 U/l), respectively (P < 0.001 for both) (Fig. 1). However, no significant differences in GGT levels were found between abstainers and former drinkers (27.0 ± 1.8; 17.5 ± 1.7 U/l).

Although not reported, we can assume that the F test for group differences, overall, was significant for both men and women. The authors then describe the results

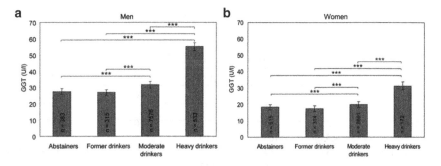

Fig. 5.3 Serum GGT as a function of drinking status, separately by gender. Reprinted with permission of Oxford University Press from Tynjala et al. (2012)

of the Bonferroni tests of mean differences. The horizontal lines over the tops of the bars in the men's and women's figures in Fig. 5.3 are designed to reveal which group means are significantly different from each other. Any group means that are not joined by a separate horizontal line are not significantly different. For example: for the men, we see the lines above the "heavy drinkers" bar join heavy drinkers with each of the other drinking groups. This means that the mean serum GGT is significantly different for heavy drinkers vs. moderate drinkers, former drinkers, and abstainers. Similarly, the bars above "moderate drinkers" join moderate drinkers with former drinkers and abstainers. Hence, moderate drinkers have mean serum GGT that is significantly different from that of former drinkers and abstainers. The two groups who are not joined by their own horizontal line are abstainers and former drinkers. These groups are therefore not significantly different in mean serum GGT. The lines in the women's figure are similarly interpreted.

χ^2: Second-to-Fourth Digit Ratio Study

The second-to-fourth digit ratio of the right hand is apparently associated with prenatal testosterone levels and prenatal estrogen (Jung et al. 2010). Jung and colleagues therefore investigated whether this ratio might predict prostate volume and PSA levels in men. Three hundred and sixty-six men presenting at a Korean hospital with lower urinary tract symptoms, aged 40 or older, and with a PSA level ≤40 ng/mL were prospectively enrolled in their study. All patients underwent transrectal ultrasonography. One analysis dichotomized second-to-fourth digit ratios as <0.950 vs. ≥0.950, producing two groups of men. These men were then compared on several dichotomized study endpoints via the χ^2 statistic. Their results are shown in Table 5.6:

What is shown in the table here are (a) the contingency tables for the association between digit ratio and binary versions of several variables of interest, (b) the p value for the χ^2 statistic for each contingency table, (c) the odds ratio (OR) for the

Table 5.6 Cross-classification of study endpoints by Second-to-Fourth Digit Ratio Group [Reprinted with Permission of John Wiley and Sons, Publishers, from Jung et al. (2010)]

		Digit ratio				
		<0.950 (Group A)	≥0.950 (Group B)	p Value	OR	95 % CI
Age (years)	≥65	82	77	0.663	1.096	0.725–1.658
	<65	102	105			
PV (cc)	≥35	79	63	0.102	1.421	0.931–2.168
	<35	105	119			
PSA (ng/mL)	≥3.0	54	35	0.024	1.745	1.073–2.838
	<3.0	130	147			
PSAD (ng/mL/cc)	≥0.10	36	23	0.072	1.682	0.952–2.971
	<0.10	148	159			
Prostate biopsy	Done	54	35	0.024	1.745	1.073–2.838
	Not done	130	147			
Cancer	Present	21	7	0.006	3.221	1.334–7.778
	Absent	163	175			
Cancer detection	Yes	21	7	0.061	2.545	0.943–6.868
	No	33	28			

Table 5.7 Crosstabulation of PSA (ng/mL) with digit ratio category; numbers in cells are observed frequency (column %) [expected frequency]

	Digit ratio		
PSA (ng/mL)	<0.950	≥0.950	Total
≥3.0	54 **(29 %)** [44.16]	35 **(19 %)** [43.68]	89 **(24 %)**
<3.0	130 **(71 %)** [139.84]	147 **(81 %)** [138.32]	277 **(76 %)**
Total	184	182	366

odds of being in the first category of the interest variable, based on having a lower, vs. a higher digit ratio, and (d) the 95 % confidence interval (CI) for that odds ratio. Let's examine one of these subtables to see how these measures are calculated. We'll look at the association between digit ratio and PSA level (Table 5.7):

We see that 29 % of the men have a PSA ≥ 3.0 if their digit ratio is under 0.95, whereas only 19 % have a PSA that high if their digit ratio is 0.95 or higher. So it looks like a lower digit ratio is associated with a higher probability of a higher PSA. The chi-squared statistic is

$$\chi^2 = \frac{(54-44.16)^2}{44.16} + \frac{(35-43.68)^2}{43.68} + \frac{(130-139.84)^2}{139.84} + \frac{(147-138.32)^2}{138.32} = 5.15,$$

which has a p value of 0.024, as is shown in Table 5.6. Moreover, the odds ratio (i.e., for the odds of having a PSA ≥ 3.0 for those with a lower, vs. a higher digit ratio) is

(0.29/0.71)/(0.19/0.81) = 1.741. In the table, it is shown as 1.745. This is due to a different way of calculating the odds ratio that avoids any rounding error: OR = (54) (147)/(35) (130) = 1.745. Hence, the odds of having a higher PSA are about 75 % higher if one has a higher (vs. a lower) digit ratio. The other significant associations in the table show that men with a lower digit ratio were also more likely to have undergone prostate biopsy and to have been diagnosed with prostate cancer.

Paired t Test: Bariatric Surgery and Urinary Function Study

Both urinary incontinence and erectile dysfunction have been found to be associated with obesity (Ranasinghe et al. 2010). Therefore, Ranasinghe and colleagues studied the effects of bariatric surgery on urinary and sexual functioning in males and females. Their retrospective study involved sending questionnaires by mail to all patients who underwent laparoscopic gastric banding surgery (LGB) between 2001 and 2009 at one particular surgical practice. Their sample consisted of 142 females and 34 males who responded to the survey. The respondents were mailed a questionnaire containing several standardized scales for detecting urinary symptoms, such as the International Consultation on Incontinence Questionnaire Short Form (ICIQ-SF) and the International Prostate Symptom Score (IPSS), and asked about their perceptions of urinary symptoms before and after surgery. They were also asked a "Quality of Life" question (p. 89): "If you were to spend the rest of your life with your urinary condition the way it is now, how would you feel about that?" It is not clear how this question is coded, however. Most likely the scores range from something like 1 for "okay" to 5 for "miserable." Counterintuitively, the higher scores represent a *lower* quality of life, as is evident in their interpretation of results (see below). On average, it had been just over two-and-a-half years since the surgery. Here is how the authors describe one type of analysis they performed (p. 89): "Paired *t*-tests were used to determine if there had been a statistically significant change in weight, body-mass index (BMI) and individual questionnaire scores after LGB." Table 5.8 shows the results of these *t* tests:

Here is how they describe the results (all *p* values in the table are for the paired *t* test). All "Change" scores are calculated approximately as mean After—mean Before:

> There was a significant weight loss in both males and females after LGB. The males had a greater weight loss than females (23.2 kg vs 22.7 kg), but females had a greater BMI loss (7.51 vs 8.28). In females, the ICQ-SF ($P = 0.0008$) and QOL ($P < 0.0001$) symptoms both significantly improved after LGB. However, there was no improvement in urinary function despite weight loss after LGB in males (Table 2).

As a final comment, we note that it would be better if the "Before" scores were actually measured prior to surgery rather than being based on recall. It's always possible that, as part of an unconscious attempt to justify having had the surgery, respondents may tend to recall their symptoms before the surgery as being worse than they actually were.

Table 5.8 Paired *t* tests for mean differences in study endpoints after vs. before LGB [Reprinted with permission of John Wiley and Sons, Publishers, from Ranasinghe et al. (2010)]

| Outcome of interest | Gender | Mean (SD) of outcomes | | | *p* |
		Before	After	Change	
Weight (kg)	Male	145.6 (28.31)	123.3 (23.19)	−23.1 (18.35)	<0.0001
	Female	118.3 (18.50)	96.7 (18.48)	−22.7 (15.74)	<0.0001
Body mass index (kg/m^2)	Male	47.3 (12.67)	38.4 (6.18)	−7.51 (5.78)	<0.0001
	Female	43.5 (6.65)	35.5 (6.80)	−8.28 (5.78)	<0.0001
ICIQ	Male	1.82 (3.43)	1.67 (3.59)	0.40 (3.55)	0.5418
	Female	5.24 (5.05)	3.93 (4.83)	−1.30 (4.34)	0.0008
Quality of life	Male	1.56 (1.52)	1.50 (1.54)	−0.06 (1.35)	0.8006
	Female	2.48 (1.94)	1.79 (1.78)	−0.72 (1.72)	<0.0001
Urinary frequency (IPSS)	Male	1.35 (1.57)	1.62 (1.69)	0.26 (0.90)	0.0951
	Female	1.60 (1.61)	1.24 (1.42)	−0.39 (1.42)	0.0032
Incomplete emptying	Male	0.53 (1.02)	0.62 (1.13)	0.09 (0.51)	0.3246
(IPSS)	Female	0.93 (1.33)	0.67 (1.05)	−0.25 (1.28)	0.0298
Nocturia (IPSS)	Male	1.88 (1.55)	1.79 (1.49)	−0.09 (0.93)	0.5851
	Female	1.98 (1.63)	1.62 (1.57)	−0.37 (1.01)	<0.0001

Fig. 5.4 Scatterplot of tumor volume against body mass index for 1,275 patients. Reprinted with permission of John Wiley and Sons, publishers from Capitanio et al. (2011)

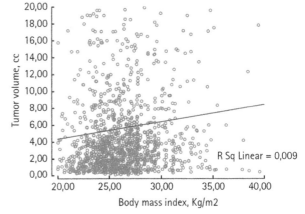

Correlation Coefficient: Obesity and Tumor Volume in Prostate Cancer

Capitanio and colleagues (2011) hypothesized that excess body weight would be associated with larger prostate tumors independent of obesity prevalence in a particular nation, race, and continent of origin. They employed data from 1,275 consecutive Caucasian prostate cancer patients treated with radical prostatectomy and pelvic lymphadenectomy at an Italian Hospital between 2006 and 2009. Among other analyses, they examined the correlation between body mass index (BMI; measured as kilograms of body weight divided by squared height in meters) and tumor volume (TV), in cubic centimeters (cc). Figure 5.4 presents a scatterplot of that relationship:

We see that a line has been drawn through the data to show the linear trend in the plot: as BMI increases, so does tumor volume. The "R Sq Linear" shown in the plot refers to r^2. The correlation coefficient is the square root of this, which is 0.095. This indicates, as is evident from the slope of the line in the plot, that there is a positive correlation between BMI and tumor volume. But the relationship appears rather weak. Is it significant? The authors have not reported that, but it's easy to calculate the t test for r here:

$$t = \frac{0.095}{\sqrt{\dfrac{1-0.095^2}{1,275-2}}} = 3.40.$$

With 1,273 df, this is very significant (one-tailed $p=0.00034$, from a Hewlett-Packard Scientific Calculator). Although the clinical significance of this relatively weak correlation may not be impressive, it is very statistically significant, due to the relatively large sample size and concomitantly enhanced power.

Preview. In the next chapter we continue the discussion of analyzing association between two quantitative variables. But instead of focusing on the correlation coefficient, we introduce the notion of a statistical model. That is, we will "model" the study endpoint as a linear function of the explanatory variable, introducing one of the most important of statistical techniques: linear regression modeling. With regression modeling, we can analyze the relationship between an explanatory variable and a study endpoint while controlling for any number of other potentially confounding variables. This vastly improves our ability to rule out latent selection bias as a problem for our analyses.

Chapter 6
Linear Regression Models

Modeling the Study Endpoint Using Regression

The correlation coefficient discussed in the last chapter is a component of one of the most important techniques in statistics: *linear regression modeling*. In this section, we introduce this topic and the subject of statistical modeling, in general. We begin with the familiar step of analyzing the association between a study endpoint and one explanatory variable, with both as quantitative variables. We then expand our model to include several explanatory variables, using the multiple linear regression model. Examples drawn from the GSS and the journal literature help to flesh out this topic.

What Is a Statistical Model?

A *model* is a set of one or more equations describing the process or processes that generated the scores on the response variable (or variables). A model is essentially a statistical conceit. We entertain the notion that the world is driven by invisible equations, and our job is to estimate them. That is, we assume that the population of scores on the response variable is determined by an equation that is "out there" in the "population," somewhere. This equation is a function of treatment as well as purely random fluctuations in human response, the latter being called *experimental error*. This is most likely not an accurate depiction of reality. However, it doesn't have to be. We are guided by the saying attributed to the statistician George Box: "All models are wrong; some are useful" (Gill 2001). To the extent that models help us understand and predict human response, they have value. In truth, all of the statistical techniques we have covered so far are underpinned by statistical models. We've just avoided cluttering the discussion with technical jargon up to now. However, understanding regression requires an understanding of modeling.

A. DeMaris and S.H. Selman, *Converting Data into Evidence: A Statistics Primer for the Medical Practitioner*, DOI 10.1007/978-1-4614-7792-1_6, © Springer Science+Business Media New York 2013

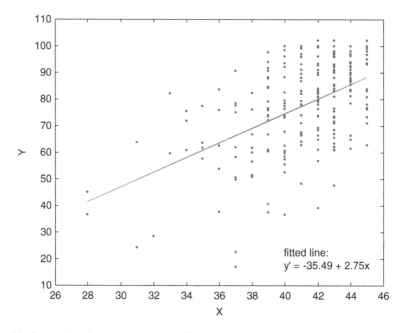

Fig. 6.1 Scatterplot of score on first exam (*Y*) plotted against math diagnostic test (*X*). Reprinted with the permission of John Wiley and Sons, Publishers, from DeMaris (2004)

A Regression Model for Exam Scores

Regard Fig. 6.1 above. It shows a scatterplot of two variables based on data collected from students in the first author's introductory statistics classes over a 10-year period. The two quantitative variables of interest are a math diagnostic test measure (*X*), based on a form administered on the first day of class, and students' scores on the first exam (*Y*), given in week 6 of the course. The math diagnostic is intended to measure math proficiency. It is believed that those with greater math proficiency tend to do better on the first exam. The reason is that statistics is a form of applied mathematics and requires the same kinds of abstract reasoning skills as math does. This is, indeed, what the scatterplot shows, as the exam scores tend to be, on average, higher, the greater the diagnostic score (the observed range of the diagnostic was from 28 to 45). The correlation between variables here is 0.52.

Linear regression modeling assumes that these data were generated, in the "population" of students taking introductory statistics, by a linear equation of the form $\mu_y = \alpha + \beta X$. The Greek letters all represent population quantities and are not directly observed. They are interpreted as follows: μ_y is the mean of exam scores for all students in the population having a particular diagnostic score, *X*. The mean of *Y* at each *X* is assumed to lie on a straight line whose equation is $\alpha + \beta X$, where α is the equation intercept—the *Y* value at which the line crosses the *Y* axis—β is the slope of the line, and X is the diagnostic score. The individual exam scores, however, do not all lie on the line. They are perturbed away from the line by random "noise," or, as we have called it above, experimental error. If the population equation is written in terms of the individual scores, Y, then it is $Y = \alpha + \beta X + \varepsilon$, where ε represents that random error. As $\varepsilon = Y - (\alpha + \beta X)$, it is clear that the error represents the difference between the actual exam score and its mean value—as represented by the line.

As we noted, our job is to estimate this equation using sample data. The technique used for estimation is called *ordinary least squares* or OLS. How does it work? The counterpart, for the sample, of the population equation is $Y = a + bX + e$, where "a" is an estimate of α and "b" is an estimate of β. Our estimate of the population mean exam score at any given diagnostic value, μ_y, is the point on the line $a + bX$, which is denoted $\hat{y}$ (called "y-hat"). That is, $\hat{y} = a + bX$. If this line is used to predict every individual Y value, we will make a series of errors in prediction, denoted e. That is, $e = Y - \hat{y}$ or $e = Y - (a + bX)$. The idea behind OLS is that the best estimate of the population line, $\alpha + \beta X$, is that line in the sample that minimizes the total error in predicting Y using the sample equation $a + bX$. Now, the errors are both positive and negative and tend to cancel each other out, so total error is measured by the *sum of the squared errors*. That is, we are looking for the a and b that minimize the sum of squared prediction errors (hence the name "least squares" in ordinary least squares). For a given sample, the X and Y values are fixed. Therefore the size of the errors only depends on the values chosen for a and b. Using calculus, it is a simple matter to find the formulas for a and b that minimize prediction error. These are then the OLS estimates of α and β.

For the current example, the "fitted line" in the lower right corner of Fig. 6.1 shows the OLS estimate of the population regression equation ($\hat{y}$ is shown as "y'" here). There are two primary benefits to be derived from the model. First, it is useful for forecasting. Suppose a prospective student is worried about his or her math ability and wants to know whether it's possible to do well in the course. I can give that person the diagnostic test and then use the diagnostic score to generate an estimated score on the first exam. The student can then judge whether this bodes well or ill for their overall performance. So if their diagnostic score were, say, 42, then their estimated score on the first exam is $-35.49 + 2.75\,(42) = 80.01$, which is a B. Not a bad performance. Second, the slope of the equation, 2.75, tells us the nature and magnitude of the effect that math proficiency has on course performance. Intuitively, each additional point on the math diagnostic is worth, on average, another 2.75 points on the exam. Thus, I can describe how the treatment affects the response in precise mathematical terms.

Other Important Features of Regression

Some nuances of regression need to be mentioned at this point. First, there are several assumptions that should be satisfied before OLS estimation of linear regression models is undertaken. We won't go into all the details, but two assumptions are especially important. One is that the model we're trying to estimate is *linear in the parameters*. What this means is that the right-hand side of the population regression equation is in the form of a weighted sum. That is, the parameters α and β are weights that multiply variables (i.e., β multiplies X) or constants (i.e., α multiplies the constant 1). The error term, ε, is an unobserved variable that is multiplied by the "parameter" 1. An equation that is *not* linear in the parameters is $Y = \alpha + X^{\beta} + \varepsilon$. Notice that this is no longer a weighted sum, since β is an exponent of X rather than being a weight that multiplies it. This equation is therefore nonlinear in the parameters and is ideal for estimating a *nonlinear relationship* (in particular, an exponential, or accelerating positive, trend) between Y and X. It can be estimated by a technique called *nonlinear least squares*. We won't cover that here. However, nonlinear models are very important and we will cover two of them in detail in Chaps. 7 and 8 (in particular, logistic regression and the proportional hazards model).

Another important assumption, known as the *orthogonality condition*, is that ε (the error term in the population regression equation) is uncorrelated with X. If this is not the case, then our estimate, b, of β will be biased. Violation of the orthogonality condition usually happens whenever an unmeasured variable in the population that is correlated with X also affects Y. (This is precisely the situation depicted in Fig. 1.1, in which health awareness was the unmeasured variable at issue.) With just one X in the model, the orthogonality condition is almost surely violated, unless there is random assignment to levels of X. Unfortunately, orthogonality cannot be verified with the data. The reason is that an artifact of OLS estimation is that e is always uncorrelated with X in the sample, making it appear that orthogonality is satisfied. (The fact that e is uncorrelated with X is very important for understanding statistical control, so let's remember this feature of OLS regression: Corr$(X, e)=0$, i.e., *the correlation between X and e is always zero*.)

The second nuance is how we evaluate the goodness of a model. The most commonly employed measure for that purpose in linear regression is r^2, which we have already encountered above. One could argue that unless a model is reasonably "good," it shouldn't be used for forecasting. For the introductory statistics example, the model r^2 is 0.268 (not shown). Recall that r^2 ranges from 0 to 1, so this represents a moderately effective model. R^2 is arguably the most cogent measure of model effectiveness. Therefore we consider it in more detail here. R^2 is referred to as a measure of *discriminatory power* (DeMaris 2004). If X has a causal effect on Y, then r^2 is essentially telling us what proportion of the variability in Y is generated by the causal effect of X. Recall that the sample regression equation is $Y = a + bX + e$. It is easily shown that the total variance in Y is equal to the variance of $(a+bX)$ plus the variance of e. That is, the total variability in Y consists of two components: the variability *of* the regression line (i.e., $a+bX$) and the variability *around* the regression line (represented by e). Figure 6.2 depicts one situation that is possible.

What is shown is the scenario in which 100 % of the variability in Y is accounted for by its regression on X (admittedly unrealistic, but useful for heuristic purposes). If we ignore X and only look at Y scores, then this two-dimensional figure is effectively collapsed to one dimension, which is the Y axis. There, we see substantial variability in Y, with Y values ranging from 1 to 21. This is the total variability in Y,

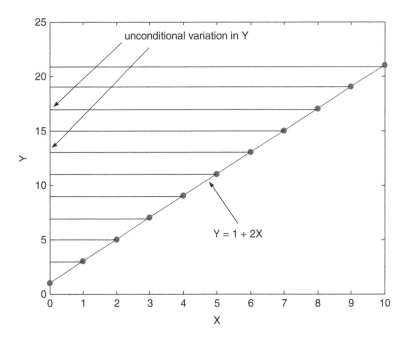

Fig. 6.2 Variability in Y completely accounted for by X. Reprinted with the permission of John Wiley and Sons, Publishers, from DeMaris (2004)

termed "unconditional variation in Y" in the figure. However, Y is perfectly determined by X via the equation $Y = 1 + 2X$. There is no experimental error. Thus, at any given X value, there is *no* variability in Y; there is just one value. For example, if X is 5, Y is 11. If X is 8, Y is 17, and so forth. This means that, at any particular X value, Y is perfectly determined: no variability in Y is exhibited. The difference between the total (or unconditional) variance in Y and the variance in Y at each X (i.e., the conditional variance in Y, given X) is what is *accounted for* by Y's regression on X. In this extreme case, *all* of Y's variability is accounted for by X, and therefore r^2 is 1. Y only exhibits variation because X is varying and "taking Y with it," so to speak. That is, all of the variability in Y is due to the fact that (a) X is varying from 0 to 10, and (b) Y values are being generated in lock-step with X. This is the extreme case of perfect determination of Y by X.

A more realistic scenario is shown in Fig. 6.3.

Here, we see that Y is no longer perfectly determined by X. The line in the middle of the points is the sample regression line: $\hat{y} = 1 + 2X$ ($\hat{y}$ is shown as y' in the figure). Although there are points that lie on the regression line, several are displaced away from the line. If we ignore X and look only at the Y scores again, the total variance in Y turns out to be 58.4. However, the variance of Y at each X value (visually revealed as the spread of the two points on either side of the line) is only 17.2. This is all of the variability in Y that remains at each X value. Now, $58.4 - 17.2 = 41.2$. So 41.2 of the total variance in Y of 58.4, i.e., 71 % of the total variance in Y, is accounted for by Y's regression on X. In this case, therefore, the r^2 is 0.71. At the

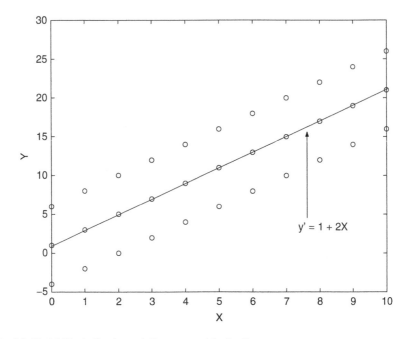

Fig. 6.3 Variability in Y only partially accounted for by X

other extreme, if the slope estimate is zero, none of the variance in Y is accounted for by X, and $r^2 = 0$. To understand why this is the case, we decompose the variance of Y in terms of the regression model (see, for example, DeMaris 2004, Chap. 3): $s_y^2 = b^2 s_x^2 + s_e^2$. That is, the variance of Y is equal to the square of the slope times the variance of X plus the variance of e. So if the slope is zero, *all* of the variance in Y is error variance, and none is generated by X. Normally, Y is partly determined by X and partly determined by random error, and r^2 nicely encapsulates the proportionate contribution of X to the variability in Y in this process.

Multiple Linear Regression

So far we have considered a regression model having only one predictor. This is known as simple linear regression or SLR. However, often we want to employ several predictors, or, especially in observational studies, we want to *control* for several other potentially confounding variables. This is accomplished with the multiple linear regression, or MULR, model. When there is more than one X in the model, the procedure is called either a "multivariate" or a "multivariable" analysis.

The MULR model for the mean of a response (or study endpoint) is

$$\mu_y = \alpha + \beta_1 X_1 + \beta_2 X_2 + \ldots + \beta_K X_K,$$

where "K" stands for the total number of predictors (or "regressors") in the model. or, in terms of an individual Y score:

$$Y = \alpha + \beta_1 X_1 + \beta_2 X_2 + \ldots + \beta_K X_K + \varepsilon,$$

where ε represents experimental error, once again. Again, ε is assumed to be purely random "noise" arising naturally from the study of human response. It is also assumed to be uncorrelated with all of the Xs in the model. This is the orthogonality assumption, again. If this condition is violated, then one of more of the sample estimates of the βs will be biased.

Statistical Control in MULR

The βs in the model are called *partial slopes* or *partial regression coefficients*. They represent the effects of each variable controlling for all of the other variables in the model. That is, β_1 is the unit change in the mean of Y for a one-unit increase in X_1, controlling for (i.e., holding constant) all of the other Xs in the model. The other βs have comparable interpretations. The concept of statistical control is so important that we will take it up at length here. There are two ways to understand statistical control. The first is more intuitive; the second is more technically accurate.

An Intuitive Sense of Control

First, then, imagine that we were able to randomly assign units to a treatment group and a control group. We'll refer to group status simply as X. We know that, through randomization, those in the two different groups would have the same average value of any third variable, Z, *which also affects Y*. This means that if the treatment has an effect on Y, it's not because of the "action" of Z on Y, since the groups are no different, on average, on Z. Thus, there is no need for statistical control over Z in this instance. In the absence of random assignment, however, the two groups would likely be different on their average level of Z. Therefore, we don't know how much it is X that affects Y, or the fact that X is related to level of Z, which, in turn, is what affects Y. How can we mimic random assignment after the fact? The closest we can come is to examine how X affects Y *among all those who have the same value* of Z. The equation that we want to estimate, then, is $Y = a + b_1 X + b_2 Z + e$, where b_1 represents the effect of X *among all those who are the same on Z*. Figures 6.4, 6.5, 6.6, 6.7, and 6.8 below show how this plays out.

What is shown in Fig. 6.4 is a bivariate scatterplot of Y against X. It looks like there's a pretty strong effect (note that a slope is also referred to as an "effect" throughout this primer) of X on Y. The slope is 1.44. However, it turns out that a second variable, Z, is partly responsible for this seemingly strong effect. Z has a

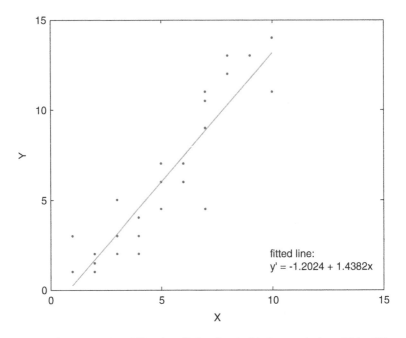

Fig. 6.4 Bivariate scatterplot of Y against X. Reprinted with the permission of John Wiley and Sons, Publishers, from DeMaris (2004)

Fig. 6.5 Relationship between X, Y, and Z that underlies Fig. 6.4

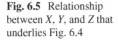

strong positive effect on Y and is highly positively correlated with X. The scenario is displayed in Fig. 6.5.

As is evident from the figure, all paths connecting the three variables are positive. This means that if Z is not controlled, i.e., if it is left out of the model for Y, the product of the positive path between X and Z with the positive path between Z and Y, the result of which is positive, will be added to the positive path between X and Y, making it appear that X has a particularly strong positive effect on Y.

Z has only three values: 1, 2, or 3. So let's examine a scatterplot of Y against X separately for all units who have the same value of Z. This way we can see how much X affects Y when Z is *held constant* (another term for statistical control). Figures 6.6, 6.7, and 6.8 show the $X-Y$ scatterplots for each level of Z.

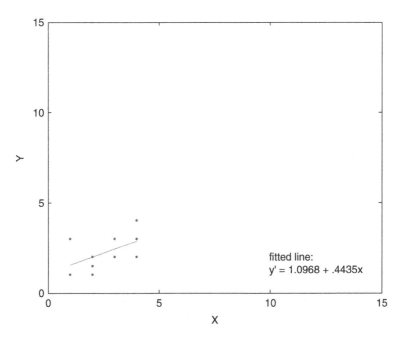

Fig. 6.6 Bivariate scatterplot of Y against X when $Z=1$. Reprinted with the permission of John Wiley and Sons, Publishers, from DeMaris (2004)

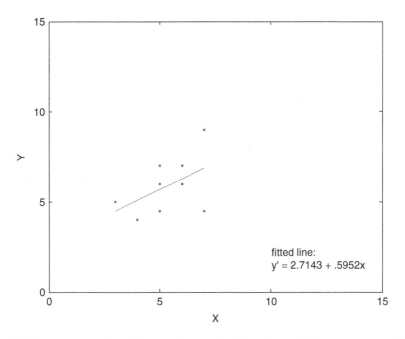

Fig. 6.7 Bivariate scatterplot of Y against X when $Z=2$. Reprinted with the permission of John Wiley and Sons, Publishers, from DeMaris (2004)

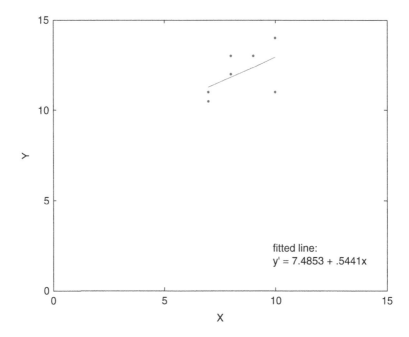

Fig. 6.8 Bivariate scatterplot of Y against X when $Z=3$. Reprinted with the permission of John Wiley and Sons, Publishers, from DeMaris (2004)

Figure 6.6 shows the scatterplot of Y against X for all the points having $Z=1$. This group of points should be recognized as the lowest third of the points in Fig. 6.4.

Figure 6.7 shows the scatterplot of Y against X for all the points having $Z=2$. This group of points should be recognized as the middle third of the points in Fig. 6.4.

Figure 6.8 shows the scatterplot of Y against X for all the points having $Z=3$. This group of points should be recognized as the highest (and rightmost) third of the points in Fig. 6.4.

What we notice in Figs. 6.6, 6.7, and 6.8 is that the slope of the line relating X to Y is now considerably reduced, compared to the slope in Fig. 6.4. This suggests that the positive effect of X on Y is substantially weaker when Z is held constant, as should obtain based on Fig. 6.5. The strong positive association of Z with Y can be seen by the fact that the cluster of Y scores moves up the Y-axis dramatically as Z goes from 1 to 2 to 3. Similarly, the strong positive association of Z with X can be seen by the fact that the clusters of points move from left to right along the X-axis as Z goes from 1 to 3. At any rate, the slope of the X effect on Y is, respectively, 0.444, 0.595, or 0.544, for $Z=1, 2, 3$. Since these values are not very different from each other, we can just average them, which gives us 0.528. We could then report 0.528 as *the* effect of X on Y *controlling for* Z. Technically, this is not completely accurate. The partial slope of X in a MULR of Y on X and Z (estimated via OLS but not shown) is 0.564 instead of 0.528. But it's close enough to convey a notion of how control is effected.

No-Interaction Assumption. It is important to notice that the slope of X in Figs. 6.6, 6.7, and 6.8 is about the same in each case. So averaging these three slopes and reporting the result as *the* effect of X on Y, controlling for Z, is pretty accurate. But what if the three slopes were very different? Suppose, for example, that they were 0.545, 0, and −0.545 for $Z = 1$, 2, and 3, respectively. Then their average is zero. In this case, controlling for Z would produce a very misleading picture. It would appear that X had absolutely no effect on Y once Z is held constant. But this is incorrect. It's just that the effect of X is very different as we go from one level of Z to another. This latter situation is called *statistical interaction*. This term means that the association between X and Y changes as we go from one level of Z to the next. When that happens, we would say that X and Z *interact* in their effects on Y or that Z *moderates* X's effect on Y. This phenomenon is a very important part of real data analysis and happens with regularity. We will take it up when we discuss the analysis of the GSS data using MULR below. In the meantime, the take-home point is that controlling for a third variable assumes that the relationship between the original two variables (i.e., X and Y) is exactly (or pretty closely) the same at each level of that third variable. If that is not the case, then we need to use an *interaction model* to analyze the data. We will see what one of these looks like below.

R^2 *for MULR.* In MULR the analogue of r^2 is R^2. This represents the variation in Y that is accounted for by *all* of the Xs in the regression together. Again, this value ranges from 0 to 1. In the artificial-data example of Fig. 6.4, the R^2 for the MULR of Y on X and Z is 0.92. With real data, one rarely sees anything so impressive.

Hypothesis Tests in MULR. Additionally, there are statistical tests of hypothesis in MULR, as in all procedures. These are typically concerned with two issues. First, is the model of any utility in predicting Y? The null hypothesis is that all of the partial regression coefficients equal zero. This is tested with an "F" test, similar to the F test in ANOVA. If that test is significant, the second issue is: which predictor effects (i.e., which partial slopes) are significant? This is addressed using a t test for the significance of each partial slope. The formula for each such test is $t = b/\text{se}$, where "b" is the partial slope in question and "se" is the standard error of that partial slope.

Statistical Control: Technical Details

We mentioned above that the averaging of the separate effects of X on Y at different levels of Z wasn't quite an accurate depiction of control. For the second perspective on control, we consider how it's accomplished mathematically. Regard Fig. 6.5 again. Suppose the figure represents a mechanical system in which the "circles" around the three variables are gears and the lines are drive shafts. And suppose the shaft from X to Y is hidden from view. If we turn the X gear the Y gear turns. But one reason is that the X gear is connected to the Z gear, so turning X turns the Z gear, which also turns the Y gear. But we want to know whether the X gear is connected directly to the Y gear, so that turning X also results in a turning of Y, independently of the link through Z. What could we do? Well, the obvious solution is to disconnect the link from X to Z. This means that Z doesn't turn when we turn the X gear. So if we turn the X gear under this condition, and the Y gear turns, then there is a connection there.

Now, let "turning" be equivalent to variation. What we need to do with X is to examine how variation in X relates to variation in Y while keeping Z from covarying (or varying along) with X. Here's how that's done. Recall that the estimated MULR equation is $Y = a + b_1 X + b_2 Z + e$. How do we actually obtain b_1, say? Recall from above that, in SLR, Corr$(X, e) = 0$. That is, the error term, e, is uncorrelated with the predictor in that equation. Therefore suppose we regress X on Z, via the equation $X = c + dZ + u$. (This is just an SLR of X on Z, where we're using different letters for intercept, slope, and error term.) Then Corr$(Z, u) = 0$. Note that u is defined as $u = X - (c + dZ)$. That is, u is a version of X from which the linear association between X and Z has been subtracted out or removed. That is, *u is a version of X that is purged of its linear association (correlation) with Z.* If we then estimate the SLR: $Y = a' + b'u$ we will see that b' here is our b_1 in the MULR. Effectively what we've done is to be able to let X vary and see how Y responds, but without Z varying at the same time. That is, it's as if Z is being held constant as X is varying, which corresponds with our intuitive understanding of control. (The same mathematical operation underlies the partial slope for Z in the same MULR.) You can imagine, however, that if X and Z are too highly correlated (say, at a level of 0.95 or more) subtracting out the linear association with Z will leave almost nothing behind. That is, u would exhibit almost no variation, because most of X's variance was accounted for (or generated) by Z. In that case, the regression of Y on u would be very unreliable, since if there's little variation in the predictor, there can't be much *co*variation with Y. The situation of X and Z being very highly correlated is known as *multicollinearity* in MULR. It is of concern because it interferes with reliable estimation of the partial slopes for variables that are affected by it. It isn't often a serious problem, but if you see a reference to that term, you'll know what's being referred to. (It's a problem that's also easily remedied most of the time via a variety of ameliorative strategies.)

An Example Using the GSS

Recall the physician stewardship variable from the 2002 GSS discussed in Chap. 4. We found that women were significantly lower on it than men were. We might ask what other factors affect physician stewardship. Or, we might speculate that, because men have, on average, greater annual income than women, they can more easily afford to use physicians' services than women can. This might be why they're more willing to "leave the driving" to their doctors, so to speak. Thus we might ask if there's still a gender difference in physician stewardship once income is held

Table 6.1 Regression results for physician stewardship

```
. regress relydoc female age educ rincom98

    Source |      SS       df       MS              Number of obs =    1769
-----------+------------------------------          F(  4,  1764) =    28.46
     Model | 338.078204     4   84.519551           Prob > F      =   0.0000
  Residual | 5238.39212  1764  2.96961004           R-squared     =   0.0606
-----------+------------------------------          Adj R-squared =   0.0585
     Total | 5576.47032  1768  3.15411217           Root MSE      =   1.7233


-------------------------------------------------------------------------------
   relydoc |     Coef.   Std. Err.       t    P>|t|     [95% Conf. Interval]
-----------+-------------------------------------------------------------------
    female |  -.508551   .0842242     -6.04   0.000    -.6737409   -.3433612
       age |  .0070189   .0031394      2.24   0.025     .0008616    .0131762
      educ | -.1103932   .0155185     -7.11   0.000    -.1408297   -.0799566
  rincom98 | -.0216513   .0078814     -2.75   0.006    -.0371091   -.0061935
     _cons |  4.885758   .2437744     20.04   0.000     4.407641    5.363875
-------------------------------------------------------------------------------
```

constant. Table 6.1 above presents the results of a multiple regression analysis of physician stewardship for the 1,769 respondents with complete data on all variables in the analysis. It uses the variables "female (coded 1 for females, and 0 for males)," "age (respondent's age in years)," "educ (respondent's education in years of schooling completed)," and "rincom98 (respondent income coded in intervals from 1 = under \$1,000 to 23 = \$110,000 or more)." The response variable is labeled "relydoc," which stands for physician stewardship. The table is the output from a popular statistical software program called Stata.

The "Coef."column shows the regression coefficients for each X in the model; the coefficient for "_cons" is the intercept. The subsequent columns present standard errors for each coefficient ("Std. Err."), t test values for testing whether each coefficient is zero in the population ("t"), the p value associated with each t test ("$P>|t|$"), and 95 % confidence intervals for each coefficient ("95 % Conf. Interval"). There is an initial F test for the model as a whole shown in the upper right part of the table. The null hypothesis for this test is that all of the effects of the independent variables—the regression coefficients—equal zero in the population. The F value is 28.46 and is very significant ("Prob > $F = 0.0000$"). This means that at least one of the variables has a real (i.e., nonzero) effect on physician stewardship in the population. The R^2 for the model, however, isn't particularly impressive. It's 0.0606, which means that only about 6 % of the variability in physician stewardship is accounted for by our model. Nevertheless, all of the explanatory variables have significant effects on the response, as can be seen from the p values. This is most likely because we have a lot of power, given that the sample size here is 1,769 respondents.

The variable "female" needs some explanation. This isn't really a quantitative variable, so you might ask how it can be in a regression model. It so happens that the coding of the variable, with females coded 1 and males coded 0, facilitates its use in regression. A variable coded this way is called a *dummy variable*. The terminology refs to the fact that the numbers "0" and "1" don't convey any quantitative information, per se. Rather, they are convenient "labels" that allow the variable to enter a regression model. When a dichotomous variable is coded this way its coefficient turns out to be the difference in the mean of the response for the group coded 1 vs. the group coded 0, controlling the other variables. So the coefficient of −0.509 for "female" is telling us that, on average, controlling for the other Xs in the model, females are about a half point lower in physician stewardship than males. This is what we saw before without controlling for any other variables. In fact, controlling for the other variables—including annual income—has made the difference slightly greater: −0.509 with controls vs. −0.433 without controls (from Table 4.1: this is the "diff" entry representing the raw mean difference between males and females in physician stewardship). Apparently, the gender difference in physician stewardship is not just an artifact of men having more money to spend on doctors. What about the other variables? The results suggest that average physician stewardship increases with age but actually declines with both increasing income and education. So much for the "more money to spend on doctors" hypothesis!

Finally, let's write out the equation for physician stewardship, as estimated using the sample data:

$$\hat{y} = 4.89 - 0.51\text{Female} + 0.01\text{age} - 0.11\text{educ} - 0.02\text{rincom98}.$$

We could use this to get an estimated physician stewardship value for a respondent of a particular demographic profile. So for a 40-year-old woman with a college degree (i.e., 16 years of education) and an annual income level of 20, her estimated physician stewardship score would be

$$\hat{y} = 4.89 - 0.51(1) + 0.01(40) - 0.11(16) - 0.02(20) = 2.62.$$

According to the way physician stewardship is coded, this translates to a response that is approximately halfway between "moderately disagree" and "slightly disagree" with the notion of relying on the doctor's knowledge rather than finding out about one's condition on one's own (see Chap. 2 for the coding of the physician stewardship variable).

ANCOVA: A Particular Type of Regression Model

As a final comment, a multiple regression analysis containing a mixture of qualitative (e.g., gender) and quantitative (e.g., age, education, income) explanatory variables, as in the above example, is also called an *analysis of covariance*, or ANCOVA. The moniker originates from experimental settings, in which interest centers on treatment-group (a qualitative factor) differences in a quantitative study endpoint while controlling for one or more quantitative "covariates," which are simply control variables. These are usually pre-randomization characteristics, e.g., pretest scores on a study endpoint, which are strongly related to the post-treatment values of the study endpoint. Including them in the model makes a more powerful test of the treatment effect because they help to minimize experimental error. ANCOVA then involves a regression model in which the study endpoint is regressed on the treatment factor plus quantitative control variables. Therefore, the term ANCOVA has come to be applied to any regression analysis in which the explanatory variables are a mixture of qualitative and quantitative factors. Typically, however, the term "analysis of covariance" is reserved for the case in which prime interest is in mean differences in the study endpoint by treatment group. It is usually of interest to examine means for each treatment group while controlling for the covariates. Analysts can then use the ANCOVA model to get predicted values for the study endpoint for each treatment group, as we did for the 40-year-old woman's physician stewardship score above, with mean values for the covariates substituted into the equation. These predicted values are then referred to as *adjusted means* on the study endpoint by treatment group, since they are the treatment group means that adjust, or control, for the covariates. (See the applications below.)

Modeling Statistical Interaction

Recall that statistical interaction is the phenomenon in which the effect of one variable on another depends on the level of a third variable. In the regression example just considered, suppose our hypothesis is that the gender difference we've observed, in which females are lower in physician stewardship than males, depends on age. Because people have more health problems as they get older, we think that the gender difference is not as pronounced among older respondents. To test this, we divide the sample by age into those who are younger than 50 (the younger group) vs. those who are 50 or older. For the 1,290 younger respondents, we regress physician stewardship on education, gender, and income (not shown). The effect of being female on physician stewardship turns out to be -0.65925 ($p < 0.0001$). This suggests, as with the entire sample, that females are significantly lower on physician stewardship than males by about two-thirds of a unit. The same regression for the 479 older respondents (again, not shown) shows the effect of being female to be -0.32027 ($p > 0.10$). Thus, among older respondents, the gender difference is no longer significant, net of controls ("net of" controls means taking the other control variables— education and income—into account). This is an example of a statistical interaction. The gender effect changes over age, with it being significant among younger respondents but not significant among older respondents.

Nevertheless, an important question needs to be answered. Is the *difference* in the gender effect for younger vs. older respondents significant? This is a subtle aspect of interaction that is often overlooked. It is common practice to split a sample by some classification factor, such as age, and then run separate regressions within each group. This is typically called *stratification* on the classification factor in medical studies, and interaction effects may be referred to as "stratification" effects. When this is done, researchers often assume that observing different coefficients for the same predictor in the different stratification groups implies that the effects of that predictor are actually different in the *population* subgroups. But sampling error is such that any time one splits the sample based on some grouping factor, and runs separate regression models, *one will inevitably get different effects for the same explanatory variables in each group*. This does not imply that the variables in question actually have different effects in the relevant population subgroups. In the current example, the fact that the gender gap in physician stewardship is different for younger and older respondents in the *sample* does not mean that the gender gap in physician stewardship is different for younger vs. older respondents *in the population*. And this principle holds even if the gender gap is significant in one subgroup (e.g., the younger respondents) but not in the other (e.g., the older respondents). What is needed is a formal test for the *difference in the gender effect* across age groups. How is this accomplished?

The Interaction Model

The procedure is simple. We simply create a dummy variable for being 50 or older (coded 0 if the respondent is under 50 and 1 if the respondent is 50 or older) called "older." We then create the crossproduct of "older" with the variable "female" (which you recall is a dummy variable for the respondent being female). That is, we literally create a new variable that is the *product* of these two dummies. The resulting model, the *interaction model*, looks like this (where "Female * Older" is the product of the female dummy variable with the "older" dummy variable):

$$\hat{y} = a + b_1 \text{Age} + b_2 \text{Female} + b_3 \text{Rincom 98} + b_4 \text{Older} + b_5 \text{Female*Older}.$$

For those who are younger (i.e., Older=0), the regression is

$$\hat{y} = a + b_1 \text{Age} + b_2 \text{Female} + b_3 \text{Rincom 98} + b_4(0) + b_5 \text{Female*}(0)$$

or

$$\hat{y} = a + b_1 \text{Age} + b_2 \text{Female} + b_3 \text{Rincom 98}.$$

which means that b_2 is the effect of being female, or the gender gap in physician stewardship, among the younger respondents.

For those who are older (i.e., Older=1), the regression is

$$\hat{y} = a + b_1 \text{Age} + b_2 \text{Female} + b_3 \text{Rincom 98} + b_4(1) + b_5 \text{Female*}(1)$$

Table 6.2 Interaction model for the interaction of gender and age on physician stewardship

```
Parameter Estimates
```

Variable	Label	DF	Parameter Estimate	Standard Error	t Value	Pr > |t|
Intercept	Intercept	1	3.67644	0.20908	17.58	<0.0001
AGE	AGE OF RESPONDENT	1	0.00735	0.00524	1.40	0.1611
female	RESPONDENT IS FEMALE	1	-0.65925	0.09908	-6.65	<0.0001
RINCOM98	RESPONDENTS' INCOME	1	-0.03919	0.00767	-5.11	<0.0001
older	RESPONDENT IS >50	1	-0.17397	0.18206	-0.96	0.3394
femold	FEMALE* OLDER	1	0.33898	0.18714	1.81	0.0703

or,

$$\hat{y} = a + b_4 + b_1 \,\text{Age} + (b_2 + b_5)\,\text{Female} + b_3 \,\text{Rincom}\,98.$$

Notice that we have grouped the two coefficients that multiply "Female" together. So the gender gap in physician stewardship among older respondents is $b_2 + b_5$. The difference in the gender gap among older vs. younger respondents is, therefore, b_5. Hence a t test for the coefficient b_5 is a test of whether the gender gap is significantly *different* among older vs. younger respondents. Table 6.2 shows the result of estimating the interaction model shown above, using the regression software in the program SAS.

The coefficients of the regression are shown in the "Parameter Estimate" column. The last variable, "femold" is the crossproduct term of "female" times "older." As we see, the gender gap among younger respondents is the coefficient for "female," which equals −0.65925. The gender gap among older respondents is the sum of this coefficient and 0.33898, the coefficient of the crossproduct term. The sum is −0.65925 + 0.33898 = −0.32027, which agrees with the gender effect among older respondents that was given above. The difference in gender effects in the two age groups is therefore 0.33898, which as is evident, has a p value of 0.0703. Thus, at the conventional alpha level of 0.05, this difference is not quite significant. So we cannot conclude that there is a real difference in the gender effect on physician stewardship for younger vs. older respondents in the population. And this obtains even though the gender gap is significant among younger respondents but not significant among the older ones, as we noted above. The bottom line is that interaction effects are tested in regression models via crossproduct terms. And if the supposed interaction, or stratification, effect has not been subjected to this kind of test, then it is not to be considered conclusive.

Repeated Measures ANOVA: Interaction in the Foreground

A Study of Depressive Symptomatology

A type of analysis that is related to MULR is repeated measures ANOVA. Recall the ANOVA technique discussed in the previous chapter. That technique was employed when examining the association between a quantitative study endpoint and a qualitative treatment with more than two categories. But suppose we have the following scenario. A team of medical researchers wants to test which antidepressant is more effective at reducing depressive symptomatology in patients. Three hundred patients presenting with depressive symptoms at a local clinic agree to be enrolled in a clinical trial. First, they are all pretested with the Center for Epidemiological Studies Depression Scale (CES-D), a widely used paper-and-pencil measure of depressive symptomatology. This instrument asks how often in the past week the subject has experienced each of 20 different symptoms. Examples are "I was bothered by things that usually don't bother me," and "I felt that I could not shake off the blues, even with help from my family or friends." Response categories are "rarely or none of the time (<1 day)," "some or a little of the time (1–2 days)," "occasionally or a moderate amount of time (3–4 days)," and "most or all of the time (5–7 days)." The codes for each response are, respectively, 0, 1, 2, and 3. The scale ranges from 0 to 60, with higher scores indicating the presence of more depressive symptomatology. The pretest score on the CES-D is the time 1 measure in the study.

Then the researchers randomly assign 100 patients each to be treated by Celexa (treatment 1) and Wellbutrin (treatment 2), vs. placebo (control condition). These patients are then followed up every 4 months for a year. On each follow-up they are given the CES-D to fill out again. This results in three more CES-D scores for each subject, which constitute the time 2, time 3, and time 4 scores. Interest centers on the extent to which the antidepressant treatments *reduce the trajectory in depressive symptoms over time*, compared to the placebo condition. In this study, *time*, which has four levels—time 1, time 2, time 3, time 4—is another qualitative factor that affects depression, in addition to treatment. The "effect" of time would be revealed by the way in which the average depression in a given treatment group changes over time. But what is expected is that the reduction in depressive symptoms over time will be greater under the two antidepressant treatments, compared to placebo. That is, the primary effect the researchers are looking for is an *interaction* between treatment and time in their effects on average depression. The means for the three groups at each time period are shown in Table 6.3.

Analyzing the Data

Repeated measures ANOVA is typically a "two-factor," meaning two explanatory variables, ANOVA. (It can have more than two factors, too, but much of the time two factors are all that are used.) This means that there are two independent variables:

Table 6.3 Mean CES-D scores by treatment group and time period for 300 subjects

Treatment	n	Time 1	Time 2	Time 3	Time 4	Mean
Celexa	100	46.1	23.9	18.5	14.3	25.7
Wellbutrin	100	45.7	28.6	23.1	19.4	29.2
Placebo	100	46.3	43.4	41.2	41.2	43.0
Mean		46.0	32.0	27.6	25.0	

treatment and time. The analysis is complicated by the fact that the same subjects are being measured at more than one time. Thus, the four CES-D scores over time for any given subject are tied together by virtue of coming from the same person. Like the paired t test example from the previous chapter, then, repeated measures ANOVA involves dependent sampling on the repeated measure. This variable is referred to as the *within-subjects* variable, because its values vary within any given subject. That is, each subject experiences all four levels of the time variable. The other variable, the treatment factor, is called the *between-subjects* variable. This is because it only varies between subjects. That is, any given subject only experiences one level of the treatment variable—they are either in one of the treatment groups or the control group. The upshot of this design is that there is typically a positive correlation between any two sets of responses pertaining to two different time periods. So CES-D scores for the 300 subjects at time 1 are positively correlated with CES-D scores for the same subjects at time 2 or time 3 or time 4, and so forth. Because of this, the standard error for testing the effect of time or the treatment×time interaction is different from the standard error for testing the treatment effect, per se.

Time, Treatment, and Treatment × Time Effects

There are three different "effects" that come out of this analysis. The time effect can be seen in the last row of Table 6.3, labeled "Mean." It is the change in average CES-D over time, ignoring treatment group. Each number is the average of the three group means for a given time period. It is evident that there is a drop in average depressive symptomatology over time, with the mean symptom level at time 1 being 46 and the mean symptom level at time 4 being 25. The treatment effect is shown by the three means in the last column of the table. It is the difference in mean CES-D by treatment group, ignoring time. Each of these means is the average of the four means over time for a given treatment condition. Hence we can see that the Celexa treatment has the lowest mean depressive symptomatology overall (25.7), and the placebo group has the highest mean overall (43.0). Nevertheless, neither of these effects is of prime interest. The focus of the study is the change in depressive symptomatology over time, and *how this differs according to treatment category*. This is best seen in Fig. 6.9, which shows the trajectory of mean CES-D over time, separately by treatment group.

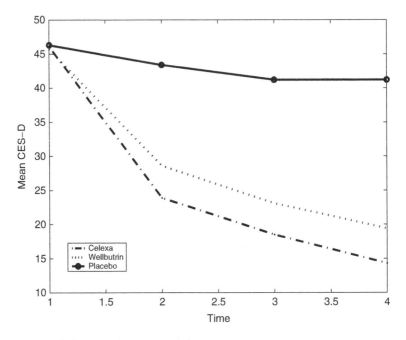

Fig. 6.9 Mean CES-D over time, separately by treatment group

It is clear in the figure, first, that mean CES-D is the same for each treatment group at time 1. This is due to the randomization, which ensures that, on average, there should be no treatment-group difference in the initial value of the study endpoint, prior to treatment. Second, it is also clear that the trajectory in average CES-D is quite different in the three groups. The Placebo group has a relatively flat trajectory, with only a slight reduction in CES-D over time. The Wellbutrin and Celexa groups, on the other hand, have much more pronounced declines in depressive symptomatology over time, with the Celexa group showing the greatest decline of the groups. Hence, as we noted at the outset, the primary effect expected in this analysis is that there would be an interaction between the two explanatory factors, treatment and time. Here we see that the interaction effect is the main "player" in the analysis.

Applications: Regression and Repeated Measures ANOVA in Action

In the following journal applications, we will see how linear regression and repeated measures ANOVA have been employed in medical research. Additionally, we will consider issues that are raised by the particular approaches taken by each research team.

Gender Difference in Physician Salaries, Revisited

Recall the study of the gender difference in physicians' salaries from Chap. 4 (Jagsi et al. 2012). Recall, also, that the mean difference in salaries between men and women physicians was $32,764 favoring the men. To what extent could this difference be explained by the fact that men had a greater number of publications and worked more hours, on average? In fact, the researchers controlled for many additional characteristics that might differentiate men and women. As reported in the article (p. 2412), there was a long list of control variables used in a multiple regression model for salary:

> We described characteristics of this sample by gender and then constructed multiple variable linear regression models for salary with the following respondent characteristics: gender, age, race, marital status, parental status, additional graduate degree, rank, leadership, specialty nature, specialty pay level, current institution type, current institution region, current institution NIH funding rank group, whether the respondent had changed institutions, K award type, years since K award, K award funding institute, receipt of R01 or greater than $1 million in grants, publications, work hours, and percentage of time spent in research.

In their regression model containing all these factors, the effect of being male on salary was 13,399 ($p = 0.001$). This means that, net of all control variables, the gender gap in average salary was still significant, amounting to $13,399.00 favoring males. The authors conclude (p. 2417):

> Ultimately, this study provides evidence that gender differences in compensation continue to exist in academic medicine, even among a select cohort of physician researchers whose job content is far more similar than in cohorts previously studied, and even after controlling extensively for specialization and productivity.

Obesity and Tumor Volume, Revisited

Recall the study by Capitanio and colleages (2011) from the previous chapter. They employed data from 1,275 consecutive Caucasian prostate cancer patients treated with radical prostatectomy and pelvic lymphadenectomy at an Italian Hospital between 2006 and 2009. Their primary interest was in examining how BMI might affect prostate tumor volume. As noted in the previous chapter, in a bivariate analysis, they found a significant, albeit small, positive correlation between BMI and tumor volume that was significant. Would this association hold up after controlling for other patient characteristics? The results of simple and multiple regression modeling are shown in Table 6.4.

The "*B* coefficient" column under "Univariable analyses" presents the regression coefficients for the simple linear regression of tumor volume ("PCa volume") on each of the predictors listed in the "Predictors" column. So the regression of tumor volume on BMI shows a regression coefficient (i.e., slope) of 0.2; the regression of tumor volume on age shows a regression coefficient of 0.02, and so forth. The "*p*" column

Table 6.4 Simple and multiple linear regression models of tumor volume based on BMI and controls [Reprinted with permission of John Wiley and Sons, Publishers, from Capitanio et al. (2011)]

Predictors	Univariable analyses		Multivariable analyses	
	B coefficient	p	B coefficient	p
BMI	0.2	0.001	0.14	0.04
Age	0.02	0.4	−0.07	0.8
Diabetes	1.41	0.05	0.87	0.3
PSA	0.11	<0.001	0.10	<0.001
Biopsy Gleason score	3.30	<0.001	2.49	<0.001
Clinical stage	3.06	<0.001	1.58	<0.001
Prostate volume	−0.01	0.5	0.07	0.4

gives p values for the test that the corresponding population coefficient equals zero, and therefore tells which of the predictors has a significant association with tumor volume. The "Multivariable analyses" columns provide the same information, but for the multiple regression of tumor volume on all seven predictors listed in the table. Hence, the partial regression coefficient for BMI in the multiple regression is 0.14, with a p value of 0.04. This is the effect of BMI on tumor volume in the multiple regression that controls for age, diabetes, PSA, biopsy Gleason score, clinical stage, and prostate volume.

Here (pp. 679–680) is how the authors describe the results in Table 6.4 (which is "Table 4" in their article):

> Table 4 shows univariable and multivariable linear regression analyses predicting TV at RP. With univariable analyses (Table 4), BMI results correlated with TV at RP ($B = 0.2$; $P = 0.001$). Moreover, PSA level, biopsy Gleason score and clinical stage were associated with cancer size at RP as well (all $P < 0.001$). Conversely, patient age and prostate volume did not predict TV at RP ($P > 0.4$). On multivariable analysis, after adjustment for age, PSA level, biopsy Gleason score, clinical stage and prostate volume, BMI reached the independent predictor status ($P = 0.04$) (Table 4).

Some commentary is in order. First, we remind the reader that "PCa" is prostate cancer, "TV" is tumor volume, and "RP" is radical prostatectomy. Second, the term "univariable" refers to the fact that the regression involves only one explanatory variable, i.e., it is simple linear regression, a form of bivariate analysis. Third, we note that the authors describe BMI results as "correlated" with TV, but then in parentheses give, not a correlation coefficient, but "B," the simple linear regression coefficient and p value for BMI. Fourth, we note that two effects that are significant in the simple linear regression either become nonsignificant in the multiple regression (i.e., diabetes—whether the patient is diabetic) or show a marked increase in p value (i.e., BMI) from the bivariate to the multivariate analysis. The reason for these changes in p values is that many of the explanatory variables are positively correlated with each other. For example, overweight people are more likely to be diabetic. Also there were positive correlations among BMI, PSA, prostate volume, and tumor grade (i.e., biopsy Gleason score). This means that the situation would be graphed as in Fig. 6.10.

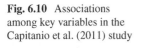

Fig. 6.10 Associations among key variables in the Capitanio et al. (2011) study

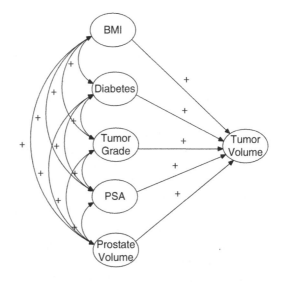

The same principle applies to Fig. 6.10 that applies to Fig. 6.5 above. That is, the simple linear regression, say, between BMI and tumor volume does not control for the other factors in the figure. Therefore all the indirect paths from BMI to tumor volume that go through the other variables are multiplied together and added to the direct path from BMI to tumor volume. This would make it appear that BMI has a particularly strong—and very significant—effect on tumor volume in the simple linear regression. In reality, that effect is the sum of many "pathways" that go from BMI to tumor volume through the other factors. This means that much of that seemingly strong "effect" of BMI in the simple linear regression is not due to BMI actually influencing tumor volume. Rather, it's the connection between BMI and these other factors, which, in turn, have influences on tumor volume, which is driving this strong effect. In the multiple regression, all these other factors are controlled. This is tantamount to severing the connections between BMI and all other factors in the diagram (the connections are all shown as curved two-headed arrows). With all those connections cut, the BMI effect is just the direct positive path from BMI to tumor volume. Although it is still significant, the force of its effect is substantially reduced. The same comments apply to the diabetes variable.

Discrimination and Waist Circumference

Hunte (2011, #25) hypothesized that interpersonal experiences of discrimination are related to an increase in waist circumference over time. The reason, according to the author, is that (p. 1233) "individuals with relatively high levels of internalized beliefs about their race/ethnicity may have adopted a defeatist mind-set, which is thought to be related to the physiologic pathway associated with excess body fat accumulation."

Hunte used the baseline (1995) and follow-up (2004) data on 1,452 respondents from the National Survey of Midlife Development in the USA. The researcher examined whether changes in the perceived experience of interpersonal discrimination had an effect on the change in waist circumference over the period. The average change in waist circumference over the 9-year period was 5.98 cm. That is, on average, respondents gained in waist size by approximately 6 cm over the period. Discrimination was assessed with a series of questions about the respondents' perception regarding how often they were subjected to various discourteous behaviors, such as being treated with less respect than other people or receiving poorer service than others. Based on these responses given at both times (1995, 2004), respondents were characterized as low stable (low discrimination at both times), decreasing (movement from higher to lower discrimination over time), increasing (movement from lower to higher discrimination over time), and high-stable (reporting high discrimination at both times) types with respect to changing discrimination over time. The analysis primarily consisted of multiple regression models in which the change in waist circumference over time (the primary study endpoint) was regressed on change in interpersonal discrimination plus several control variables. One of the controls was the respondent's waist circumference at baseline (i.e., in 1995). Results for both men and women respondents are shown separately in Table 6.5.

The results are separated by gender because Hunte found an interaction between gender and discrimination in their effects on change in waist circumference. This means that the effect of change in discrimination on change in waist circumference was significantly different for men and women, which justifies separate regression models by gender. Hunte explains this as follows (p. 1236):

> The 2-way interaction terms between sex and change in interpersonal discrimination variable were significant after adjusting for none of the covariates ($P < 0.05$) and were marginally significant ($P = 0.067$) when adjusting for all of the covariates listed in Table 2, suggesting that the relation between the change in interpersonal discrimination variable and waist circumference may differ for men and women (data not shown). Results from the sex-stratified analyses predicting mean change in waist circumference are presented in Table 2.

The explanatory variables "Decrease," "Increase," and "High Stable" shown in the leftmost column of the table are all dummy variables. Each one contrasts a particular discrimination group with the low-stable group. Accordingly, "Low stable" is listed as the "(referent)" category with a coefficient of 0.0. This notation means that "Low stable" is not actually an independent variable in the model. A variable with four categories needs only three dummy variables to represent it in the model. This is the same principle we saw with the dummy variable "female" in the model in Tables 6.1 and 6.2 above: a variable with two categories needs only one dummy to represent it in the model. Hunte describes the results in Table 6.5 as follows (p. 1236):

> These results suggest that men who consistently reported high levels of interpersonal discrimination over the study period experienced a larger (2.39 cm) increase in waist circumference compared with men who consistently experienced low levels of interpersonal discrimination ($P < 0.05$). Likewise, the waist circumference of women who reported an increase in interpersonal discrimination increased approximately 1.88 cm more than that for women who were in the low-stable group ($P < 0.05$).

Table 6.5 Regression of change in waist circumference on change in perceived discrimination plus controls [Reprinted with permission of Oxford University Press from Hunte (2011)]

	Men			Women		
	Model 1[a]	Model 2[b]	Model 3[c]	Model 1[a]	Model 1[b]	Model 1[c]
Low stable[d] (referent)	0.0	0.0	0.0	0.0	0.0	0.0
Decrease[e]	0.20 (0.82)[f]	0.20 (0.82)	0.20 (0.82)	1.57 (1.09)	1.59 (1.10)	1.54 (1.09)
Increase[g]	0.18 (0.62)	0.18 (0.62)	0.17 (0.62)	2.14 (0.88)**	2.09 (0.89)**	1.88 (0.89)**
High stable[h]	2.41 (0.96)**	2.41 (0.96)**	2.39 (0.96)**	2.27 (1.19)*	2.25 (1.19)*	2.09 (1.19)*
p Value for linear effect	>0.05	>0.05	>0.05	<0.05	<0.05	<0.05
Adjusted R-squared value	0.437	0.437	0.438	0.410	0.408	0.412
F-test result	44.764	33.901	28.746	45.747	34.361	29.533
p Value for model significance	0.0000	0.0000	0.0000	0.0000	0.0000	0.0000
No. of participants	678	678	678	774	774	774

*$p<0.10$; **$p<0.05$

[a]Adjusted for age, race discrimination at wave I, waist circumference at wave I, body mass index at waves I and II, education at wave I, household income at wave I, and depression disorder at wave I
[b]Adjusted for the covariates in model 1 and smoking at wave I, drinking at wave I, and physical activity at wave I
[c]Adjusted for the covariates in model 2 and major life events at wave II
[d]Low levels of perceived interpersonal discrimination in waves I and II; no change
[e]Change from high levels of interpersonal discrimination in wave I to low levels in wave II
[f]Values in parentheses, standard errors
[g]Change from low levels of interpersonal discrimination in wave I to high levels in wave II
[h]High levels of perceived interpersonal discrimination in waves I and II; no change

We notice here that the researcher is reporting the effects for high stable (for men) or increase (for women) categories of change in discrimination in Model 3, only, for either gender. This is because these are the "full" models for either gender, that is, the models with all possible controls in them (the controls in each model are explained in footnotes a, b, and c). Hence we see that the partial regression coefficient for High stable for men is 2.39, which is significant at $p<0.05$. This means that, on average and net of controls, perceiving high discrimination at both time periods is associated with 2.39 cm higher waist size, compared to the men in the low stable group. For women, the same discrimination variable is associated with 2.09 cm higher waist size. But this effect is only marginal; it does not reach the conventional 0.05 significance level. On the other hand, the coefficient for Increase does attain $p<0.05$ for women and suggests that those perceiving increasing discrimination over time gained in waist size by 1.88 cm, on average, compared to women in the low-stable group.

One could argue that low-stable, decrease, increase, and high-stable categories of changing discrimination constitute increasing degrees of severity of discrimination. Why not just code these values as 1, 2, 3, and 4 and enter this as just one explanatory variable in the regression? In fact, this is what the researchers did and reported as a test for a "linear trend" (p. 1236):

> The P values from the regression analyses testing for a linear trend of the interpersonal discrimination variable are presented in Tables 2 and 3. The P values suggest a positive association between interpersonal discrimination and increases in waist circumference for women but not for men over the 9-year study period (P < 0.05).

The p values resulting from these tests for a linear trend for men and women are shown in the row of values corresponding to "p value for linear effect" in Table 6.5. What these results mean is that one could, in fact, code discrimination 1–4 for women, as described above, and its regression coefficient would be positive and significant in the model when coded that way. On the other hand, if one used the same discrimination coding for men, the variable would not be significant that way. Examining the coefficients for the discrimination categories in Model 3 for women, it's clear that each higher severity of discrimination is associated with a larger effect, with the coefficients for Decrease, Increase, and High stable being 1.54, 1.88, and 2.09, respectively. But for men, this is not the case, with the coefficients being 0.20, 0.17, and 2.39, respectively. Because the 1–4 coding is not therefore sensible for both men and women, the researcher has elected to present the dummy-coded discrimination results in the table.

We notice in the table that the researcher has presented an "Adjusted R-squared value" for each model. This is comparable to the R^2 discussed above. However, it has been adjusted because R^2 tends to be a little too generous in assessing a model's predictive performance. For example, R^2 cannot possibly decrease when additional explanatory variables are added to a model, no matter how insignificant they are. For this reason, there is a corrected R^2 called the *adjusted* R^2, as is shown here. This measure has the property that it can decrease as one adds irrelevant predictors to the model. The fact that it does not decrease for the men's models suggests that successive controls added to the models were all at least reasonably important. Such is not exactly the case for the women, since the adjusted R^2 drops from 0.410 to 0.408 from Model 1 to Model 2. However, it goes back up again to 0.412 for Model 3. In terms of indicating the models' discriminatory power, the adjusted R^2 is interpreted just like R^2. Hence, about 41–43 % of the variability in change in waist circumference is accounted for by the predictors in men's and women's models. Notice, also, that at the bottom of the table the researcher presents the "F-test result," along with "p value for model significance." This is the test for overall model utility that was discussed above. Apparently, all models show a highly significant F test result, which justifies testing the individual coefficients in each model.

Reducing Alcohol Dependence: An Example of ANCOVA

Cobain and her colleagues (2011) investigated whether brief interventions delivered by a nurse specialist to nontreatment-seeking alcohol-dependent patients in a hospital setting would be effective in reducing alcohol consumption and dependence. The study was conducted at two different hospitals in England in 2007. The study was not a randomized trial. Rather, one hospital was designated the test (i.e., intervention) site and the other the control site. Patients were screened for eligibility for the study with the Alcohol Use Disorders Identification Tool (AUDIT). These scores had a range of 16–40, with mean baseline scores of 33.68 and 29.74 for the intervention and control groups, respectively. If they scored sufficiently high on this paper-and-pencil instrument, they then completed the Severity of Alcohol Dependence Questionnaire (SADQ). These scores had a range of 5–60, with mean baseline scores of 38.56 and 35.63 for the intervention and control groups, respectively. Patients receiving a positive score on the SADQ were then invited to be in the study (Cobain et al. 2011). Participating patients at the test site were given a brief intervention program by an Alcohol Specialist Nurse (ASN). This consisted of a 15–20 min session described as follows (p. 435), where "BI" represents brief intervention:

> In the intervention group, an ASN delivered BI of 15–20 min based on a commonly utilized strategy for the delivery of BI (FRAMES: feedback, responsibility, advice, menu of strategies, empathy and self-efficacy) (Bien et al., 1993). The most important element in our use of this model is the exploration of patients' perceptions of the link between their alcohol consumption and their emergency department attendance or hospital admission. There was no predetermined number of treatment sessions. Nurses made a clinical judgment of how many times a further follow-up appointment should be offered. BI took place on each follow-up appointment. The nurses suggested that patients consider a range of options for additional support, including alcohol-specific support such as Alcoholics Anonymous (AA), or other community support groups. Pharmacological adjunct therapy was not prescribed, but information was sometimes given on effectiveness and side effects so that patients could, if they wished, discuss that information with their general practitioner. There were four ASNs at the test site, and patients who attended for follow-up may have seen a different nurse at each occasion.

Participating patients at the control site simply received normal clinical care, along with advice regarding community-based services. Based on statistical power considerations it was determined to recruit 100 patients for each study group.

A follow-up interview was given to all recruited patients 6 months after their original assessments. At that time patients once again filled out the AUDIT and SADQ questionnaires regarding their alcohol dependence and provided other information, such as the number of days on which they drank, the number of drinks per day, and so forth. The statistical analysis consisted of an analysis of covariance, looking for a significant mean group (intervention vs. control) difference in several measures at the follow-up survey, with special attention to AUDIT and SADQ scores. Covariates used in the models as controls included baseline AUDIT and SADQ scores. This analysis was accomplished simply by regressing each study endpoint (e.g., AUDIT score, SADQ score, etc.) on a dummy variable for treatment group (intervention vs. control), baseline audit score, and baseline SADQ score. The results

Table 6.6 ANCOVA results for brief intervention and control groups, controlling for baseline AUDIT and SADQ scores [Reprinted with permission of Oxford University Press from Cobain et al. (2011)]

	Mean				
	Intervention ($n=48$)	Control ($n=50$)	Adjusted mean difference	95 % CI	p-Value
SADQ	12.23	30.76	−23.47	−29.76, −17.18	<0.0001
AUDIT	13.50	24.90	−15.71	−20.46, −10.96	<0.0001
No. of units per drink day	8.08	23.00	−17.51	−23.03, −11.99	<0.0001
No. of drink days	3.69	5.62	−2.55	−3.68, −1.42	<0.0001
Length of stay in hospital	2.27	4.72	−1.74	−5.26, 1.79	0.3310
No. of A&E attendances	0.71	1.82	−1.09	−2.21, 0.03	0.0572

are presented in Table 6.6. It is evident that means on SADQ, AUDIT, Number of units per drink day, and no. of drink days, at follow-up, were significantly different for intervention vs. control groups, adjusting for initial AUDIT and SADQ scores.

Here is how the authors describe the results (p. 436):

> Alcohol consumption and alcohol dependence measures (AUDIT and SADQ) at follow-up and adjusted mean differences between two treatment arms are shown in Table 2. Patients in the intervention group had significantly lower (P < 0.0001) SADQ scores than patients in the control group. SADQ scores were 23 (95 % CI 17, 30) points lower in the intervention arm. Daily consumption of alcohol and number of drink days were significantly lower (P < 0.0001) in the intervention group.

Interaction 1: Evaluating the Six-Minute Walk in MS

There is considerable interest in applying walking-performance tests as clinical outcomes in MS (Motl et al. 2012). Walking performance among MS patients is a key outcome variable that is associated with disease progression, independence, quality of life, and activities of daily living. One such promising walking test is the six-minute walk (6MW). Motl and his colleagues examined the pattern of change in cadence and oxygen consumption over the course of the 6MW among MS patients characterized by varying degrees of disability. The goal was to verify that the 6MW could serve as a good diagnostic tool for differentiating levels of disability in people with MS. The sample consisted of 95 people with clinically definite MS recruited via referrals from neurologists. All subjects completed the 6MW, which consisted of walking as far and as fast as possible for 6 min. Study endpoints were cadence in steps per minute and oxygen consumption (V·O2) in milliliters per minute. MS patients were divided into three disability levels based on their scores on the Expanded Disability Status Scale (EDSS). Disability status was classified as mild, moderate, or severe.

The researchers described their statistical strategy as follows (p. 3): "We examined differences in cadence and V·O2 over the 6MW using two-way group by time ANOVA." Although not explicitly stated, this is a repeated-measures ANOVA. The between-subjects factor was disability status. The within-subjects factor was walking

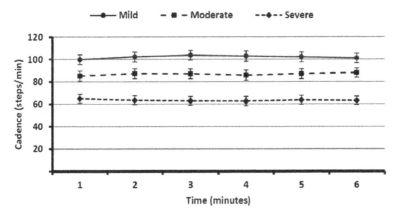

Fig. 6.11 Disability-group differences in cadence over the 6MW. Reprinted from Motl et al. (2012) from *BMC Neurology*, an open-access journal

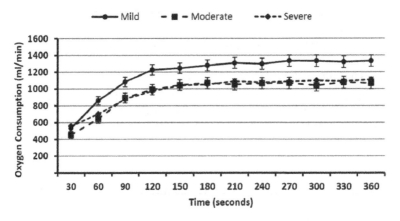

Fig. 6.12 Disability-group differences in oxygen consumption over the 6MW. Reprinted from Motl et al. (2012) from *BMC Neurology*, an open-access journal

time ranging from 0 to 360 s. The primary results are displayed in Figs. 6.11 and 6.12. Figure 6.11 shows differences in cadence in the 6MW by disability status:

The authors describe these results as follows (p. 3):

> There was a strong group main effect on cadence (steps/minute) during the 6MW, $F(2,91)$ = 22.82, p = .0001, η^2 = .33. Those with mild disability took significantly more steps per minute during the 6MW than those with moderate (d = 0.66) and severe (d = 1.64) disability, and those with moderate disability took significantly more steps per minute during the 6MW than those with severe disability (d = 0.99). This is illustrated in Figure 1. Cadence did not differ over the 6MW by time, $F(5,455)$ = 0.42, p = .84, η^2 = .01, or group and time, $F(10,455)$ = 1.08, p = .37, η^2 = .02.

The symbols "η^2" and "*d*" represent *effect sizes* and indicate how strong each effect in the analysis is. The η^2 values are like R^2s, while the *d* values represent standardized mean differences. For the η^2 values, small, moderate, and large effects are indicated by values of 0.01, 0.06, and 0.14, respectively. For the *d* values, small, moderate, and large effects are indicated by values of 0.2, 0.5, and 0.8, respectively. The group main effect on cadence had an η^2 of 0.33. This means that the group effect explained 33 % of the variance in cadence. The very low readings of the other two η^2 values suggest that the time effect and the group by time effect were very weak. All of the mean differences in cadence between disability groups had large effect sizes (0.66, 1.64, and 0.99), hence group differences in cadence were quite pronounced. The "strong group main effect on cadence" is easily seen by the different heights of the "curves" for each disability group in the figure. The fact that each curve is relatively flat and shows almost no change in elevation over time is reflected in the statement "Cadence did not differ over the 6MW by time." Similarly the statement that cadence did not differ over "group and time" refers to the fact that there was no interaction between disability status and time in their effects on cadence. This is evident in the fact that the three curves for the three disability groups are virtually parallel. This means that disability-group differences in average cadence did not vary by time. The three "*F*" values reported in the authors' statement are significance tests for, respectively, a disability-status effect (which was very significant), a time effect (which was not significant), and a group×time interaction effect (which was not significant).

Figure 6.12 shows disability-group differences in oxygen consumption over the 6MW:

Here is how the authors describe the pattern in Fig. 6.12 (p. 3):

> There was a very strong time main effect on V·O2 during the 6MW, $F(11,1012) = 357.58$, p = .0001, $\eta^2 = .80$, as well as a moderate group main effect, $F(2,92) = 4.41$, p = .015, $\eta^2 = .09$, and a moderate group by time interaction, $F(22,1012) = 4.66$, p = .0001, $\eta^2 = .09$. Overall, V·O2 increased significantly every 30 seconds over the first 3 minutes of the 6MW, and then remained stable over the second 3 minutes of the 6MW; this is illustrated in Figure 2. The overall pattern of change in V·O2 over the 6MW was not changed in additional analyses that controlled for the presence/absence of disease- modifying or symptomatic therapy. The rate of increase in V·O2 was steeper in those with mild disability than those with moderate and severe disability based on the interaction, and those with mild disability had a higher rate of V·O2 than those with moderate and severe disability based on the group main effect.

This time there is a significant disability status *x* time interaction effect, as noted by the authors ($F = 4.66$, $p = 0.0001$). This is evident in the different shapes of the curves between about 30 and 150 s. Those with mild disability have a noticeably steeper rise in V.02 consumption than those with either moderate or severe disability. On the other hand, the increase in V.02 consumption for the moderate and severe disability groups appears to be comparable.

Interaction 2: Randomized Trial of Methods of Nephrostomy Tract Closure

Li and his colleagues (2010) employed a randomized trial to evaluate three different methods of nephrostomy tract closure after percutaneous nephrolithotripsy. In the authors' words, the goal of the study was as follows (p. 1660):

Table 6.7 Repeated-measures ANOVA results for post-surgical pain [Reprinted with permission of John Wiley and Sons, Publishers, from Li et al. (2010)]

Time point	Nephrostomy tract closure method		
	Floseal, $N=3$	Fascial stitch, $N=5$	Cope loop, $N=5$
After surgery	8.3±8.7	21.8±6.8	20.8±6.8
1-week follow-up	17.0±5.5	19.2±4.3	4.6±4.3
1-month follow-up	12.3±9.7	20.0±7.5	8.6±7.5
3-month follow-up	6.7±8.8	18.6±6.8	5.4±6.9
Repeated measures of ANOVA	Degrees of freedom (df)	F-ratio (F)	p
Time	3,30	2.37	0.09
Time-by-group interaction	6,30	2.86	0.03

In this study, we performed a prospective randomized trial comparing the control group, where nephrostomy tract closure using 10-F Cope loop nephrostomy tube was used, with tubeless nephrostomy closure, where either a deep fascial stitch or a gelatin matrix haemostatic sealant (FloSeal, Baxter Medical, Fremont, CA, USA) was used. We looked for differences in perioperative variables, postoperative discomfort and complication rates.

Between April 2005 and March 2009, 31 patients undergoing percutaneous nephrolithotomy (PCNL) were randomly assigned to one of three groups: nephrostomy tract closure with FloSeal, fascial stitch, or Cope loop. Two of the primary study endpoints were a visual analog pain scale, scored 0–10, with ten representing the worst pain, and a quality-of-life measure (QOL), scored 0–100, with 100 representing the highest quality of life (Li et al. 2010). The pain and QOL scales were administered on postoperative day 1, and again at 1 week, 1 month, and 3 months after surgery. Here is how the authors describe their statistical analysis, with "SF-36" scores being the QOL scale:

> To further identify differences in the progression of SF- 36 scores and analogue pain scale, data were analysed using a repeated measures ANOVA test with four time points (within groups effect) and three surgical groups (between group effect) (Tables 2a, 3a).

As is evident, the authors performed a repeated-measures ANOVA with the treatment-group factor as the between-subjects factor and time as the within-subjects factor. The results for the pain scale are shown in Table 6.7.

In the bottom panel of the table there are two F tests shown. One is for the main effect of time, and it is not quite significant ($p=0.09$). The other is for the time x group interaction effect, and it is significant at $p=0.03$. The latter effect suggests that the trend in pain over time is different, according to surgical group. These differences are evident in the means shown in the three columns. Each surgical-group's column presents the four mean scores on pain over the time periods, plus and minus their standard errors. However, let's just regard the means. What we notice is that pain decreases quickly for the Cope loop group but much more slowly for the fascial

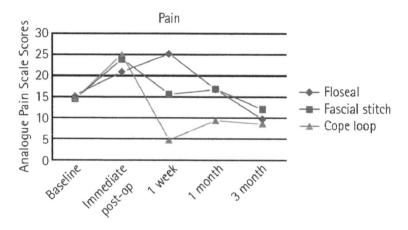

Fig. 6.13 Trends in analog pain scores for different surgical groups over time. Reprinted with permission of John Wiley and Sons, Publishers, from Li et al. (2010)

stitch group. The FloSeal group shows an increase in pain from after surgery to the 1 week follow-up, before decreasing again at 1 and 3 months after surgery.

This interaction effect is especially evident in Fig. 6.13, which shows surgical-group differences in the trajectory of analog pain scores over time. The figure shows an additional pain measurement: a baseline pain measure taken prior to surgery. Due to random assignment to surgical groups, the baseline pain scores are the same for all three groups. The aforementioned interaction effect is easily discerned from the different trends in pain over time for the three surgical groups, from "Immediate Post-op" through "3 month," and echoes the patterns shown by the means in Table 6.7.

Interaction 3: The Effect of Testosterone Treatment on Aging Symptoms in Men

Interested in countering the effect of declining testosterone levels on aging men's quality of life, Ho and colleagues (2011) undertook a randomized study to assess the effects of testosterone treatment. The primary study endpoint was the Aging Male Symptom (AMS) scale. This is a paper-and-pencil instrument that measures the severity of perceived complaints on each of 17 items tapping psychological, somato-vegetative, and sexual domains of daily life. The range of scores is 17–85, with higher scores reflecting more severe symptomatology (Ho et al. 2011). Participating males were recruited via phone-call invitation from a cohort of randomly selected men aged 40 or older from an urban Malaysian community. Inclusion criteria were age 40–70 years, having total AMS scores >27, having early morning total testosterone level <12 nmol/L on two occasions, and having a PSA level of <4 ng/mL (Ho et al. 2011,

Table 6.8 Repeated-measures ANOVA results for testosterone treatment groups [Reprinted with permission of John Wiley and Sons, Publishers, from Ho et al. (2011)]

AMS score	Intervention group	Baseline	Week 18	Week 48	Repeated measure ANOVA, F
Mean (SD) total	Placebo	38.46 (11.85)	34.66 (10.06)	33.59 (10.69)	4.576
AMS sum score	Testosterone undecanoate	41.73 (12.73)	32.73 (9.71)	32.61 (9.67)	
Mean (SD)	Placebo	10.03 (3.98)	8.88 (3.38)	8.81 (3.30)	3.922
psychological domain score	Testosterone undecanoate	11.11 (4.30)	8.61 (3.41)	8.27 (3.05)	
Mean (SD)	Placebo	15.93 (5.34)	14.58 (4.58)	14.12 (5.05)	26.174
somatovegetative score	Testosterone undecanoate	17.18 (5.52)	13.43 (4.67)	13.89 (4.48)	
Mean (SD) sexual	Placebo	12.49 (4.29)	11.20 (3.42)	10.66 (3.95)	2.512
domain score	Testosterone undecanoate	13.45 (4.34)	10.70 (3.63)	10.45 (3.69)	

p. 261). Sample size was 56 in the treatment group and 58 in the control group. The treatment and control conditions are described by the authors (p. 262):

> All participants received five injections from the package allocated to them at weeks 0, 6, 18, 30 and 42 after formal enrolment. The active treatment was 1000 mg of testosterone undecanoate in 4 mL of castor oil, and placebo was just castor oil of the same volume and appearance. The injection was given as slow bolus i.m. at the gluteal region over 1 min.

The primary study endpoint was health-related quality of life (HRQoL), as measured by the AMS score. The authors describe their statistical analysis as follows (p. 262):

> The effects of active treatment on HRQoL scores were estimated using repeated measure ANOVA by including the intervention × time interaction terms. The two-sided level of significance (P) was set at 0.05. Data analysis was done using the Statistical Package for the Social Sciences (SPSS Inc., Chicago IL, USA) version 15.

We note, once again, that a repeated-measures ANOVA is being employed to analyze the data. The authors are using the SPSS software, another popular statistical package. Table 6.8 shows the repeated-measures ANOVA results, along with mean total AMS scores and mean AMS scores for each domain of the AMS, by treatment status and time. Note that the F tests shown are all for the treatment group × time interaction effect.

Here is the authors' description of the findings in this table (p. 263):

> The improvement in the total AMS score was significantly greater in the treatment arm compared with the placebo arm (F: 4.576, df = 2.000, $P = 0.017$) over the 48-week period (Fig. 3). The change in mean total AMS score was − 12.6% in the placebo group and − 21.9% in the testosterone undecanoate 1,000 mg group. Similarly, over the 48-week period, the mean AMS psychological and somatovegetative domain scores decreased significantly more in the testosterone undecanoate 1,000 mg arm than in the placebo arm (− 2.8 vs − 1.2, $P = 0.03$ and − 3.2 vs − 1.8, $P = 0.016$, respectively), but there was no significant difference in the change in sexual subscale scores between the two groups (Table 2).

Consistent with the authors' report here, we can see that mean AMS from baseline to week 18 to week 48 shows a greater decline for the testosterone undecanoate group than for the placebo group, whether the total AMS score is considered, or the AMS psychological or somatovegetative domain scores are considered. The treatment-group difference in the pattern of change in the mean AMS scores in the sexual domain is not quite significant. The authors conclude that long-acting testosterone undecanoate treatment shows promise for improving aging men's quality of life.

Interaction 4: Spousal Support and Women's Interstitial Cystitis Syndrome

Ginting and her colleagues (2010) draw on a transactional model of health to examine how a husband's support might mitigate the impact of pain due to interstitial cystitis/painful bladder syndrome (IC/PBIS) on women's quality of life. Their focus is on the interaction between husband support and IC/PBIS in their effects on women's quality of life (HRQL, or health-related quality of life). In the authors' words (p. 714):

> Thus, the aim of the present study was to determine if spousal support influences the association between pain and patient adjustment variables (i.e. HRQL, depressive symptoms and disability) in women suffering from IC/PBIS. Given the novel and exploratory nature of the present study, no specific predictions were made.

Ninety-six women with a clinical diagnosis of IC/PBIS were recruited by letter invitation from three North American health centers. The women were asked about their experience of pain, along with how often their spouse responds in specific ways to their complaints of pain. Here is how the authors describe their statistical analysis:

> To determine whether or not spousal responses influenced the relationship between pain and patient outcomes (i.e. interaction models), data were analysed using the repeated measures general linear model (GLM) procedure. The within-subjects factor (or repeated measure) was outcome and consisted of physical HRQL, mental HRQL, disability, and depressive symptoms. Pain (SF-MPQ), solicitous spousal responses, distracting spousal responses and negative spousal responses were included in the model as covariates. To determine whether or not spousal responses influenced the relationship between pain and the outcome variables, the model included two-way interaction terms involving pain and each of the spousal response variables.

This description requires some interpretation. First, the within-subjects factor, unlike the other repeated-measures ANOVAs that we've examined, is not time. Instead, it is study endpoint. That is, each respondent is measured on four study endpoints: physical HQRL, mental HQRL, disability, and depressive symptoms. As these measures are all from the same subject, they constitute dependent sampling. They are therefore treated the same statistically as if they were, say, the same variable measured at four different times. Second, although this study involves repeated

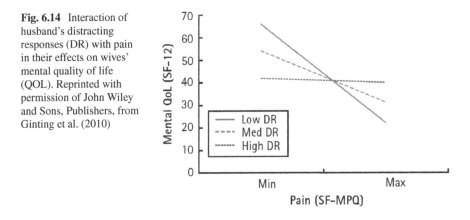

Fig. 6.14 Interaction of husband's distracting responses (DR) with pain in their effects on wives' mental quality of life (QOL). Reprinted with permission of John Wiley and Sons, Publishers, from Ginting et al. (2010)

measures, it's not an ANOVA. Notice, for example, that there is no treatment group as a between-subjects factor. One might have classified these women into different groups based on the nature of the support given to them by their husbands. If that had been the case, spousal support would have been the between-subjects factor. But instead, levels of different types of spousal support, along with pain, are included as quantitative covariates. Also included are the interactions (i.e., cross-product terms) between pain and each type of spousal support. In essence, each study endpoint (e.g., physical HQRL) is being regressed on pain, types of spousal support, and their interactions. The complication is that each study endpoint is correlated with the others, so that these regression equations are not independent. This mutual dependence among the study endpoints is taken account of in the analysis.

A primary finding was the significant interaction between pain and distracting spousal responses to wives' pain in their effects on wives' mental HQRL. Distracting spousal responses refer to the degree to which husbands try to distract wives from their pain when they complain of it. Husbands were classified into three groups based on how much they employed distracting behaviors: high-level distracters, moderate distracters, and low distracters. What the authors found was that the relationship between pain and mental HRQL was not significant for wives whose husbands were high distracters. For wives whose husbands were moderate distracters, the relationship was significant (regression coefficient for pain $= -0.66$, $p < 0.05$) but was significantly *weaker* than for wives whose husbands were low distracters (regression coefficient for pain $= -1.25$, $p < 0.05$). The authors conclude that "spousal responses may reduce or buffer the impact of pain on mental HQRL" (p. 715). Figure 6.14 illustrates this interaction finding.

What we see is that when husbands are high-level distracters (flat line in middle of graph), the slope of the linear regression of mental QOL on pain is approximately zero; i.e., pain has no effect on mental QOL. But when husbands are either moderate (dashed line) or low (solid line) distracters, the slope becomes increasingly negative. That is, greater pain is associated with lower mental QOL.

At this point, the reader should be thoroughly acquainted with linear regression and the related technique of repeated-measures ANOVA. All the techniques covered in this chapter are appropriate when the study endpoint is a quantitative variable. But what happens if the study endpoint is qualitative, and, in particular, a binary variable? It turns out that it is still possible to employ linear regression for these types of study endpoints. But the procedure is not optimal. In the next chapter we learn why and undertake the study of one of the most important techniques in the medical researcher's toolkit: logistic regression modeling.

Chapter 7
Logistic Regression

Linear regression is a widely applicable modeling tool, but it is not appropriate when the correct model should be nonlinear in the parameters. Such is the case when the study endpoint is a binary variable. The model becomes nonlinear because what is being modeled is the probability that a case experiences the event of interest or that a case is in a particular category of the binary response. As a probability must fall between 0 and 1, the linear regression model cannot accommodate it. In this chapter, we examine this important principle, develop the logistic regression model as an alternative, and consider several examples of this modeling strategy from the research literature.

Logistic Regression Model

Often the study endpoint of interest is a binary outcome, for example, whether or not a man's PSA level exceeds 4.0 or whether the result of a prostate biopsy is positive or negative for cancer. When the endpoint is binary, a linear regression model is no longer optimal. Let's consider why. Recall that a linear regression model for the population of units with, say, two regressors for simplicity, takes the form:

$$\mu_y = \alpha + \beta_1 X + \beta_2 Z.$$

Now, in the case of a binary response, Y takes on only two values, which can be represented as 1 if the unit experiences the event of interest and 0 otherwise. The mean of Y is then a proportion; in particular, the proportion of cases experiencing the event of interest in the population, or the *probability* of experiencing the event of interest. Let's let P represent that probability. Then the linear regression model becomes

$$P = \alpha + \beta_1 X + \beta_2 Z.$$

A. DeMaris and S.H. Selman, *Converting Data into Evidence: A Statistics Primer for the Medical Practitioner*, DOI 10.1007/978-1-4614-7792-1_7,
© Springer Science+Business Media New York 2013

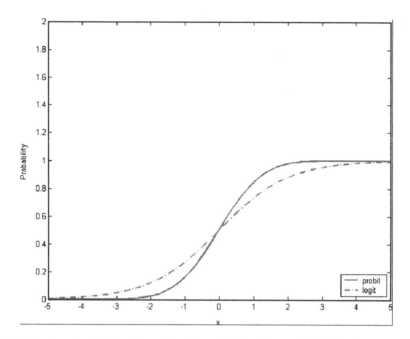

Fig. 7.1 Logit and probit functions giving the probability that a variable "*x*" takes on specific values. Reprinted with permission of John Wiley and Sons, publishers, from DeMaris (2004)

One could estimate such a model with OLS, but it's not the best strategy. The primary problem is that the right-hand side (rhs) of this equation is misspecified. The reason is that a probability has to be within the range 0–1, but the rhs of this equation is not constrained to produce only that range of values. It's entirely possible to get estimated probabilities <0 or >1 with this model. Therefore, a better approach is to find a function for the rhs that is also constrained to stay between 0 and 1. There are two such functions, and they are depicted in Fig. 7.1. The plots show how a probability is related to a single variable, *x*, through these functions.

We see here that, instead of the probability having a linear relationship to *x*—as would be true of the linear regression function—its curve is S shaped, always remaining within the bounds of 0 and 1. The solid line is for the *probit* function, which is used in probit regression, and the dashed line is for the logit function, which is used in logistic regression. We focus only on the logit function in this primer, as it is the preferred technique in medical research for a binary study endpoint. The probit function is used extensively in other fields, such as economics and other social sciences. However, as we shall see, the logit function lends itself to the interpretation of explanatory variable effects in terms of "odds ratios," which is intuitively appealing. The probit function does not have this property. Substantively, however, both modeling techniques result in the same conclusions about the sign and significance of explanatory variable effects on the study endpoint (DeMaris 2004).

The logistic regression model for a probability, as a function of two regressors, is

$$P = \frac{\exp(\alpha + \beta_1 X + \beta_2 Z)}{1 + \exp(\alpha + \beta_1 X + \beta_2 Z)}. \tag{7.1}$$

The rhs here is the algebraic formula that produces the dotted curve in Fig. 7.1 (except the curve in Fig. 7.1 only uses x, rather than $\alpha + \beta_1 X + \beta_2 Z$). In the event that "exp" is not familiar: "exp()" refers to the *exponential function*. "Exp(a)" means to raise Euler's constant to the value of a. Euler's constant is approximately equal to 2.72. For example, $\exp(2)$ is $2.72^2 = 7.398$. Euler's constant has a considerable amount of importance in both calculus (Anton 1984) and statistics (DeMaris 2004). The natural logarithm is the inverse function for the exponential function. The natural logarithm of a is the number we have to raise Euler's constant to in order to get a. For example, $\ln(7.398) = 2$ because $2.72^2 = 7.398$. Moreover, $\exp(\ln(a)) = a$ and $\ln(\exp(a)) = a$. Hence, the natural logarithm and exponential functions go hand in hand.

Because the rhs of (7.1) is a complex nonlinear function, it's not very easy to interpret the βs to describe how the regressors affect the probability. But the model can be transformed into a more interpretable version by applying the *logit transformation* to both sides of the equation. The logit transformation of the left-hand side is: $\ln[P/(1-P)]$, where "ln" refers to the natural logarithm (I use "log" interchangeably with "ln" in this primer). Substituting the rhs of (7.1) in place of P in the logit transformation gives us the transformation for the rhs of the equation in (7.1). The result is the logistic regression equation:

$$\log\left(\frac{P}{1-P}\right) = \alpha + \beta_1 X + \beta_2 Z. \tag{7.2}$$

The expression inside the parentheses, $P/(1-P)$, is the *odds* of event occurrence. The odds is just the ratio of two probabilities. (Recall that, although it seems grammatically incorrect, the odds is treated as singular.) In this case it's the ratio of the probability the event occurs to the probability it does not occur. The odds is intuitive for most people. For example, 2-to-1 odds, or an odds of 2, indicates that the event is twice as likely to happen as not. This means that the probability of event occurrence must be 0.667, since $0.667/0.333 = 2$. The left-hand side of (7.2) is therefore the log of the odds (or *log-odds*) of event occurrence. The rhs is the same as in linear regression. So the βs are interpretable as the change in the log-odds per unit increase in a given regressor, holding the other regressor constant. This still isn't entirely satisfactory, since it's hard to get a feeling for what a change in the log-odds means. Therefore, we can write the equation yet once more, in terms of the odds itself:

$$\frac{P}{1-P} = \exp(\alpha + \beta_1 X + \beta_2 Z). \tag{7.3}$$

Now, let's consider what happens to the odds if we increase X by one unit while holding Z constant:

$$\frac{P}{1-P}\Big|_{x+1} = \exp(\alpha + \beta_1(X+1) + \beta_2 Z) = \exp(\alpha + \beta_1 X + \beta_2 Z)\exp(\beta_1). \quad (7.4)$$

What happens is the original odds (which equals $\exp(\alpha + \beta_1 X + \beta_2 Z)$) gets multiplied by $\exp(\beta_1)$. Therefore, we can say that each unit increase in X, holding Z constant, magnifies the odds by $\exp(\beta_1)$. This provides a convenient way to describe how each independent variable affects the odds of event occurrence. We just exponentiate the relevant regression coefficient to find the magnitude of the (multiplicative) change in the odds for a unit increase in the regressor. $\text{Exp}(\beta_1)$ is called the *odds ratio* (since it's the ratio of the odds in (7.4) to the odds in (7.3), above) and is often the preferred way of presenting logistic regression results.

Estimation of Logistic Regression Coefficients

Logistic regression models are not estimated with OLS. Instead, we use one of the most important estimation techniques in statistics: *maximum likelihood estimation*. The way this works is as follows. For any unit sampled from the population, we can express the probability that $Y = 1$ for that unit as

$$P(y = 1) = P^y(1-P)^{1-y}.$$

This is called the *Bernoulli* probability distribution function. So, for that unit, the probability that his or her y is 1 is $P^1(1-P)^{1-1} = P$. And the probability that his or her y is 0 is $P^0(1-P)^{1-0} = 1-P$. The formula just expresses those probabilities in a compact form. Note that P varies over cases, since people's risks for an event vary from person to person. Now, the probability that we get a particular collection of ones and zeros for our Ys in any sample is just the product of all those Bernoulli functions over all of the sample cases (this is the same principle we use to figure the probability of getting three heads in a row in three coin tosses: it's $(0.5)(0.5)(0.5) = 0.125$). That joint probability is

$$P(\mathbf{y}) = \prod P^y(1-P)^{1-y}. \quad (7.5)$$

where $P(\mathbf{y})$ here represents the probability associated with the complete collection of ones and zeros in the sample, and the large "π" indicates the multiplication together of several terms. The function in (7.5) is called the *likelihood function* for the logistic regression model. Recall that P is a function of the regressors and their effects (i.e., the βs), as shown in (7.1) above. So, substituting (7.1) for P in (7.5) makes it clear that (7.5) is a complex function of the βs. In fact, once the sample has been gathered, the Xs and Ys are fixed. So $P(\mathbf{y})$ in (7.5) is then only a function of α

and the βs. In maximum likelihood estimation, we choose as values for the α and the βs those values that maximize the likelihood function. These are then the parameter values that would have made the researcher's sample of Ys *most likely to have been observed* (hence the name "maximum likelihood"). The estimation process is an iterative scheme in which a series of successive approximations is used to find the solution to a collection of nonlinear simultaneous equations. When this solution is found, the parameter estimates can then be plugged back into (7.5) to arrive at an estimated likelihood or probability of observing the sample Ys. This is sometimes reported in logistic regression results in log form, i.e., one may see "log likelihood" reported in a logistic regression table. However, this quantity is of no particular interest in and of itself and can be safely ignored.

An Example

Recall the 2002 GSS data used to illustrate multiple linear regression in the previous chapters. In that same survey, respondents were asked about whether or not they had health insurance. Figure 7.2 shows how the question was presented and coded, along with the responses for 2,755 respondents giving valid responses to the question.

Here, "IAP" means inapplicable. We see that the vast majority of respondents—86.6 %—have health insurance. Only 13.4 % of respondents do not have health insurance. (Ten respondents said either that they did not know whether they had health insurance or gave no answer to the question.) What kinds of people don't have health insurance, then? To find this out, we can perform a logistic regression using this variable as the study endpoint. However, we will recode it so that 1 = no health insurance and 0 = has health insurance. The new variable is called "uninsured." Also, we only use the 1,773 respondents who had valid data for all variables in the analysis. The results are shown in Table 7.1.

HLTHPLAN	R HAD MEDICARE OR MEDICAID		
Description of the Variable			
855. Do you have any health insurance, including Medicare or Medicaid?			
Percent	**N**	**Value**	**Label**
86.6	2,387	1	YES
13.4	368	2	NO
	52,322	0	IAP
	7	8	DONT KNOW
	3	9	NO ANSWER
100.0	55,087		**Total**

Fig. 7.2 Distribution of insured status for GSS respondents

Table 7.1 Logistic regression of uninsured status on explanatory variables in the GSS

Predictor	b	SE(b)	Exp(b)	z	p value	95 % CI
Intercept	2.3205	0.4394	–	5.2811	<0.0001	–
Age	−0.0278	0.0057	0.9730	−4.8772	<0.0001	(0.9620–0.9830)
Female	−0.5581	0.1521	0.5720	−3.6693	0.0002	(0.4250–0.7710)
Education	−0.1265	0.0277	0.8810	−4.5668	<0.0001	(0.8350–0.9300)
Income	−0.0967	0.0132	0.9080	−7.3258	<0.0001	(0.8850–0.9320)
Black	0.0250	0.1980	1.0250	0.1263	0.8994	(0.6960–1.5120)
Other race	0.7558	0.2383	2.1290	3.1716	0.0015	(1.3350–3.3970)
Model χ^2	161.2327				<0.0001	
Df	6					
H-L χ^2	12.1883				0.1430	
Df	8					
Pseudo R_1^2	0.1041					
Pseudo R_2^2	0.2004					

The table shows the explanatory variables used in the model ("Predictor"), the regression coefficients ("b"), the standard errors of the regression coefficients ("SE(b)"), the exponentiated regression coefficients ("Exp(b)"), the test statistic for testing whether each regression coefficient is significant ("z"), the p value for the test statistic ("p value"), and a 95 % confidence interval for the exponentiated regression coefficients ("95 % CI"). Four decimal places are used throughout so that some of the example computations can be illustrated. In the bottom half of the table, beginning with "Model χ^2," are several measures of the goodness of the model that will be explained below.

Interpreting the Coefficients

Several of the individual coefficients are significant. Thus we see that older respondents, women, the more educated, and those with more income are all less likely to fall into the uninsured category. Compared to Whites, however, those of other races than Black (the "Other race" variable) are more likely to be uninsured. On the other hand, Blacks are no different from Whites in the probability of being uninsured, controlling for other factors in the model. The "Exp(b)" column converts the coefficients into odds ratios for easy interpretation. Thus, each additional year of education magnifies the odds of being uninsured by a factor of 0.881. To express this in terms of a percent change in the odds, we use the transformation $100 \times [\exp(b) - 1]$. That is, each year of education reduces the odds of being uninsured by about $100 \times [0.881 - 1] = -11.9$, or 11.9 %. The odds of being uninsured for those of other races is 2.129 times greater than the odds for Whites. Or, the odds of being uninsured for those of other races is $100 \times [2.129 - 1] = 112.9$ % greater than for Whites. The other odds ratios are similarly interpreted.

Predicted Probabilities

Suppose we would like to get the estimated probability of being uninsured, based on the model, for a particular profile of person: a 25-year-old male of race other than Black or White, with a high-school education and average income (mean income is 13.773 here). Here's how we go about it. First, let's get the estimated log-odds of being uninsured for this person by evaluating the equation using their characteristics:

$$\text{Log } (P/(1-P)) = 2.32 - 0.028(25) - 0.558(0) - 0.127(12) - 0.097(13.773) + 0.756(1) = -0.484.$$

Then this person's estimated odds of being uninsured is obtained by exponentiating this result:

$$\text{Exp}(-0.484) = 0.616.$$

Finally, the estimated probability of being uninsured is just the odds divided by one plus the odds:

$$P = 0.616/(1 + 0.616) = 0.381.$$

Hence, according to the model, this person has about a 38 % chance of being uninsured.

Test Statistics and Confidence Intervals

Maximum likelihood estimation assumes that one's sample size is reasonably large. Under that condition, the regression coefficients have a normal distribution. Therefore the test statistic for testing whether each regression coefficient is significant is a z test, just like the test statistic for testing that the population mean is a particular value from Chap. 3. That is, for any regression coefficient, b, the hypothesis is that the corresponding population regression coefficient, β, is zero. Since b is normally distributed we need to find out how many standard deviations b is away from zero so we can know how discrepant the sample results are from what we would expect under the null. The "standard deviation" in question is the standard error of the coefficient, i.e., SE(b). So the test statistic is a z test of the form:

$$z = \frac{b-0}{SE(b)} = \frac{b}{SE(b)}.$$

That is, the test statistic is just the ratio of the coefficient to its standard error. For example, from Table 7.1, the test for whether the effect of age is significant is $z = -0.0278/0.0057 = -4.8772$, with a p value that is <0.0001. It is, indeed, very significant. The other z test statistics for the other coefficients are calculated in the same manner.

The confidence intervals in the column "95 % CI" are arrived at using the standard errors of the coefficients, along with the knowledge that the coefficients are normally distributed. Because each coefficient is normally distributed, adding and subtracting 1.96 standard errors from it gives us a 95 % confidence interval for the coefficient. For example, a 95 % confidence interval for the coefficient for being female is $-0.5581 \pm 1.96(0.1521) = (-0.8562, -0.2600)$. This means we are 95 % confident that the effect of being female (vs. being male) on the log odds of being uninsured is between -0.8562 and -0.2600. This can easily be converted into a confidence interval for the odds ratio [Exp(b)] by exponentiating both values. Thus $\exp(-0.8562) = 0.4250$, and $\exp(-0.2600) = 0.7710$, which agrees with the confidence interval shown in the table.

There is also a global test for the utility of the model in logistic regression. This is comparable to the overall F test in linear regression discussed in the previous chapter. If this is significant, then at least one of the coefficients of the regression in the population is nonzero, and we then use the z tests discussed above to discern which these are. The global test for logistic regression, however, is not an F test. Rather it is a chi-squared test and is called the *Model Chi-Squared Test* (or the *Likelihood-Ratio Chi-Squared Test*) and is denoted "Model χ^2" in Table 7.1. As is evident, the test is very significant ($p < 0.0001$), suggesting that the model is of some utility in predicting uninsured status.

Examining Model Performance

Although a model may be of some utility in predicting the study endpoint, we may want to know, in particular, *how much* utility. There are various ways of assessing the model's "fit" to the data or the model's "predictive utility." DeMaris (2004) has labeled model fit *empirical consistency*. This refers to the extent to which the study endpoint "behaves" the way the model says it should. On the other hand, he labels predictive utility *discriminatory power*. This property refers to the extent to which the model is able to separate, or discriminate, different cases' statuses on the study endpoint from each other. Here we discuss measures of both empirical consistency and discriminatory power for the logistic regression model.

Hosmer–Lemeshow Chi-Squared Test. Define a "case" as a subject experiencing the event of interest and a "control" as a subject who does not experience the event. A widely used test of empirical consistency for the logistic regression model is the Hosmer–Lemeshow test (Hosmer and Lemeshow 2000). The idea behind this measure is to use the chi-squared statistic to compare the observed frequencies of cases and controls in the sample with their expected values under the model. With quantitative variables in a logistic regression model, however, each subject typically has a unique predicted probability of being a case. This means that there are as many different predicted probabilities of being a case as there are subjects in the sample. It might seem reasonable to compare whether subjects really are cases with these

Table 7.2 Deciles of risk and Hosmer–Lemeshow chi-squared test of empirical consistency

Partition for the Hosmer and Lemeshow Test

Group	Total	Uninsurd = 1		Uninsurd = 0	
		Observed	Expected	Observed	Expected
1	177	7	4.78	170	172.22
2	177	4	7.79	173	169.21
3	177	7	10.62	170	166.38
4	177	10	13.12	167	163.88
5	177	16	16.08	161	160.92
6	177	21	19.75	156	157.25
7	177	30	24.48	147	152.52
8	177	36	31.38	141	145.62
9	177	50	42.09	127	134.91
10	180	60	70.92	120	109.08

Hosmer and Lemeshow Goodness-of-Fit test

Chi-square	DF	Pr > ChiSq
12.1883	8	0.1430

probabilities, however, this cannot be done using a chi-squared test. In order to maintain the properties necessary for the statistic to have a chi-squared distribution, subjects are grouped into categories based on their predicted probabilities of being a case. In particular, *deciles of risk* are formed based on the predicted probabilities of being a case. Group 1 consists of the $n/10$ subjects with the lowest probabilities, group 2 the $n/10$ subjects with the next-lowest probabilities, and so on, up to group 10, which consists of the 10 % of the sample with the highest predicted probabilities. Let $\hat{P}$ equal the predicted probability of being a case, according to the model. Once the 10 groups have been identified, the expected number of cases in each group is calculated as the sum of $\hat{P}$ over all subjects in that group. Similarly, the expected number of controls is the sum of $(1 - \hat{P})$ over all subjects in the same group. The Hosmer–Lemeshow statistic is then the chi-squared statistic for the resulting table of observed and expected frequencies. Under the null hypothesis that the model is empirically consistent, this statistic has a chi-squared distribution with 8 degrees of freedom. A significant χ^2 implies a model that is *not* empirically consistent. Table 7.2 shows the deciles of risk and the ensuing Hosmer–Lemeshow chi-squared test for empirical consistency for the logistic regression model in Table 7.1. This table was produced by the SAS software program.

The table shows the deciles as the "Group" column. The first decile, consisting of 177 subjects, is the group with the lowest risks of being uninsured, according to the model. It has 7 observed cases and 170 observed controls. According to the model, the expected number of cases for this group is 4.78, and the expected number of controls is 172.22. The other deciles all have higher risks of being uninsured, culminating in Group 10, the highest decile of risk, with 180 subjects. For this group, there were 60 observed cases and 120 observed controls. The expected number of cases and controls in this group, according to the model, are 70.92 and 109.08, respectively. The Hosmer–Lemeshow statistic is shown at the bottom of the table as 12.1883. It is not significant ($p = 0.1430$). This means that the expected numbers of cases and controls (according to model predictions) are not very different from the actual numbers of cases and controls. And this suggests that the model is indeed empirically consistent or has an acceptable fit to the data. This statistic is also reported in the bottom half of Table 7.1 as "H-L χ^2." However, an empirically consistent model may not have much predictive power, as the following discussion reveals.

Pseudo-R^2 Values. In multiple linear regression, the most commonly used measure of discriminatory power is R^2. In logistic regression, because of the binary nature of the study endpoint, calculating an R^2 measure is far more complicated. Many counterparts to R^2 have been proposed for use in logistic regression (see, for example, Long 1997), but no single measure is consistently used. Additionally, many of these do not have the same interpretation as in linear regression. Although they typically range from 0 to 1, they cannot be interpreted as the variance in the study endpoint explained by the model. In an extensive simulation, DeMaris (2002) investigated the performance of eight popular pseudo-R^2 measures for logistic regression. The two best-performing measures are shown in Table 7.1 as "Pseudo R_1^2 " and "Pseudo R_2^2." An advantage to these two measures is that both of them do have an explained-variance interpretation. However, they differ as to what the study endpoint represents. Pseudo R_1^2 (referred to as "explained risk" and denoted "$\hat{\Delta}$" by DeMaris) assumes that the study endpoint is a true qualitative difference in state. In this example, that's reasonable. Either one has health insurance or one does not. A woman is either pregnant or she is not. And so forth. Pseudo R_1^2 is then interpreted as the variation in the event in question that is accounted for by the logistic regression model. In the current example, it's telling us that about 10 % of whether or not one has health insurance is explained by the model. Pseudo R_2^2, on the other hand (called the "McKelvey-Zavoina R^2" and denoted "R_{MZ}^2" by DeMaris), is more appropriate when the binary study endpoint is a crude proxy for a quantitative underlying variable. For example, suppose we are studying depressive symptomatology. Subjects have all taken the CES-D and have a score on depressive symptomatology as a result. But the only information retained for them is whether or not their score was >25, a threshold deemed the cutoff for being clinically depressed. So all we have recorded on subjects is a binary indicator of whether or not they are clinically depressed. In a logistic regression of this binary indicator on a set of predictors, our interest might be in how the predictors influence depressive symtomatology per se, not just whether someone is clinically depressed. In that case, we might want to estimate the variance explained by our model in the quantitative underlying variable of depressive symptomatology. Pseudo R_2^2 would be the measure to use for this. Thus, if whether or not one has health insurance were a proxy for a quantitative measure of the *extent* of health insurance, say, then Pseudo R_2^2 is telling us the model explains about 20 % of the variance in that underlying measure. As a final note, neither Pseudo R_1^2 nor Pseudo R_2^2 is a routine part of the

Table 7.3 Classification table for being uninsured, based on logistic regression model in Table 7.1

Classified	Observed status		Total
	Insured	Uninsured	
Insured	1,519	223	1,742
	99.2 %	**92.5 %**	
Uninsured	13	18	31
	0.8 %	**7.5 %**	
Total	1,532	241	1,773
	86.4 %	**13.6 %**	
Criterion	0.50		
Sensitivity	7.5 %		
Specificity	99.2 %		
False positive rate	0.8 %		
Percent correctly classified	86.7 %		
Percent correct by chance	76.5 %		

output of statistical software. For this reason, they are not yet commonly used. So if the reader sees a "Pseudo R^2" measure reported for logistic regression, he or she should not assume that it has an explained-variance interpretation.

The ROC Curve. Another way to examine discriminatory power for the logistic regression model is to examine how well it allows us to correctly classify subjects with respect to the study endpoint. This is assessed in the following manner. Obtain the model-predicted probabilities of experiencing the event for each subject, in the manner illustrated above for our 25-year-old male. If that probability is greater than some criterion value, typically taken to be 0.50, classify that subject as a case. If the probability is below the criterion, classify that subject as a control. Then compare the model-based classification to the subject's actual status on Y to see how well the model leads to correct prediction of the subject's status on Y. Repeat this operation for all the subjects in the sample. Table 7.3 shows the result of this process for the logistic regression model in Table 7.1.

We see that, of 241 uninsured cases in the sample, 18 or 7.5 % were correctly classified as uninsured by the model. The probability of a case being classified by the model as a case is called the *sensitivity* of classification; therefore sensitivity is 7.5 % for this model. On the other hand, the probability of a control being classified by the model as a control is called the *specificity* of classification. In this example, 1,519 out of 1,532 controls were correctly classified as controls. Therefore, specificity is 99. 2 %. One minus the specificity is the *false positive rate*, i.e., the probability of a control being mistakenly classified by the model as a case. In this instance, that is 0.8 %. To the extent that sensitivity is greater than the false positive rate, as in this instance, the model has value. The probability of a case being classified as a case is greater than the probability of a control being classified as a case. On the whole, however, the model doesn't appear to perform all that well, which is also consistent with the relatively low pseudo-R^2 values in Table 7.1. In all, 1,519 insured subjects

Table 7.4 Classification table for being uninsured, based on logistic regression model in Table 7.1

	Observed status		
Classified	Insured	Uninsured	Total
Insured	1,431	190	1,621
	93.4 %	**78.8 %**	
Uninsured	101	51	152
	7.6 %	**21.2 %**	
Total	1,532	241	1,773
	86.4 %	**13.6 %**	
Criterion	0.30		
Sensitivity	21.2 %		
Specificity	93.4 %		
False positive rate	6.6 %		
Percent correctly classified	83.6 %		
Percent correct by chance	76.5 %		

were correctly classified as "insured" by the model, and 18 uninsured subjects were correctly classified as "uninsured." That means that $(1,519 + 18)/1,773 = 0.867$ or 86.7 % of the cases are correctly classified by the model. However, fully 76.5 % would be correctly classified just by chance alone. But most of the errors in classification are for cases. Perhaps classification performance of the model can be improved by setting the criterion lower.

Table 7.4 shows the results of setting the criterion at 0.30 instead of 0.50.

What this table shows is that sensitivity has been improved, but at the cost of specificity. Sensitivity is 21.2 % but specificity has dropped to 93.4 %. Nevertheless, sensitivity is higher than the false positive rate of 6.6 % But the percent correctly classified has also dropped some to 83.6 %. We notice, however, that we are not misclassifying the cases as badly as we were in Table 7.3, so there appears to be some improvement in that regard.

Since the sample percent uninsured is only 13.59 %, why not try that value as the criterion? Table 7.5 shows this result.

Once again, we have improved sensitivity at the expense of specificity, with both values now approximately the same—69.7 % and 69.5 %, respectively. And we note that sensitivity is more than twice as great as the false positive rate, as well. However, this time only 69.5 % of cases are correctly classified, which is actually worse than we could do by chance alone! Nevertheless, the accuracy of classification of both cases and controls appears to be strongly affected by choice of criterion value.

The idea of varying the classification criterion—as in Tables 7.3, 7.4, and 7.5—gives rise to the *receiver operating characteristic*, or ROC, curve. The idea is to vary the criterion incrementally from 0 to 1, each time generating a classification table such as Tables 7.3, 7.4, and 7.5. Afterwards, a plot of sensitivity against the false positive rate, based on the entire collection of classification tables, produces the ROC curve. This is shown in Fig. 7.3 for the model in Table 7.1.

The area under the curve, or AUC, is the key measure of interest. (This is also called the "concordance index" or the "C" statistic.) It is interpreted as the *likelihood*

Table 7.5 Classification table for being uninsured, based on logistic regression model in Table 7.1

	Observed status		
Classified	Insured	Uninsured	Total
Insured	1,065	73	1,138
	69.5 %	**30.3 %**	
Uninsured	467	168	635
	30.5 %	**69.7 %**	
Total	1,532	241	1,773
	86.4 %	**13.6 %**	
Criterion	0.1359		
Sensitivity	69.7 %		
Specificity	69.5 %		
False positive rate	30.5 %		
Percent correctly classified	69.5 %		
Percent correct by chance	76.5 %		

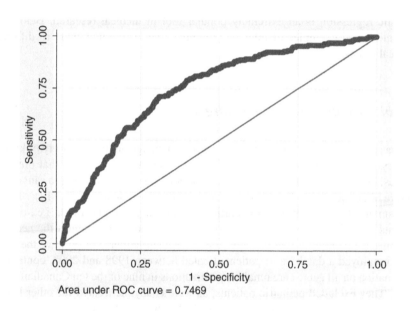

Fig. 7.3 ROC curve for logistic regression model of uninsured status in Table 7.1

that a case will have a higher predicted probability of the event than a control across the range of criterion values investigated. The diagonal line in the middle of the graph represents an AUC of 0.50. This is the minimum AUC a model could demonstrate and would suggest a model of absolutely no discriminatory power. AUC values above 0.7 generally indicate models with acceptable discriminatory power, with higher AUCs implying even better performance. For example, an AUC above 0.80 is considered "excellent," and an AUC above 0.90 is "outstanding"

(Hosmer and Lemeshow 2000). The AUC for the model of uninsured status in Table 7.1 is 0.75, which is just in the adequate range, but not great. This suggests that the model needs improvement before it would be useful for forecasting.

As a final comment, it should be noted that logistic regression is also used when the study endpoint has more than two categories. If these categories represent a qualitative variable, the procedure is then called *multinomial logistic regression*. If the categories represent rank order on some attribute but there are not enough categories to treat the response as a quantitative variable for linear regression, then the technique is called either *ordered logit modeling* or *ordinal logistic regression*. These variants on the logistic regression model see extensive use in the social and behavioral sciences, but are not often employed in medical research.

Applications: Logistic Regression in Action

Logistic regression is an extremely popular tool in medical research. Below we present several examples of interesting applications of the technique to different medical issues.

Morbidity Following Kidney Surgery

Abouassaly et al. (2011) studied the effect of patient age on the morbidity of kidney surgery associated with renal cell carcinoma. They were concerned that previous studies, largely based on single-institution populations, have painted too sanguine a picture about outcomes for this patient population. In their words (p. 812): "Better assessment of surgical morbidity, particularly in those at highest risk, i.e., elderly patients, would allow better preoperative counseling and may suggest the need for less invasive therapy in these groups, e.g., active surveillance or ablative therapy." They employed a database of patients treated between 1998 and 2008, containing information on all acute care renal hospitalizations in nine of the ten Canadian provinces. They excluded pediatric patients, as well as anyone treated for other than a solid or cystic renal mass, leaving a total of 24,578 patients for analysis. Explanatory variables included patient age, Charlson score (a measure of comorbidity), year (coded as fiscal year category), surgeon and hospital volumes for kidney procedures (both coded in quartiles), and patient income level (coded in quintiles). The study endpoint for the logistic regression was the probability of the patient having any complication after surgery. Table 7.6 is a partial reproduction of their logistic-regression results table (results for complications after partial nephrectomy as another study endpoint, as well as some covariates, are not shown).

The results shown here are for the case of radical nephrectomy surgery. Notice that all effects are for qualitative factors, represented as sets of dummy variables. There is just one *p* value reported in the column "Overall *p* Value" for each qualitative factor. This *p* value tells us whether that qualitative factor, per se, has a significant

Table 7.6 Logistic regression analysis of predictors of complications after radical nephrectomy (RN)

	RN*	
	OR (95 % CI)	Overall p Value
Age category		<0.0001
Less than 50	Referent	
50–59	0.98 (0.88–1.08)	
60–59	1.14 (1.03–1.25)	
70–79	1.39 (1.26–1.53)	
80 or greater	1.74 (1.52–1.98)	
Charlson category		<0.0001
0	Referent	
1	1.88 (1.73–2.05)	
2	3.57 (3.19–4.00)	
3 or greater	6.22 (5.18–7.48)	
Fiscal yr category		<0.0001
1998–1999	Referent	
2000–2001	0.99 (0.90–1.09)	
2002–2003	1.04 (0.94–1.15)	
2004–2005	0.95 (0.86–1.05)	
2006–2007	0.68 (0.61–0.75)	
Surgeon vol quartile		<0.0001
Low	Referent	
Intermediate	0.83 (0.77–0.91)	
High	0.76 (0.69–0.83)	
Very high	0.82 (0.74–0.91)	
Hospital vol quartile		<0.0001
Low	Referent	
Intermediate	1.02 (0.94–0.91)	
High	1.41 (1.28–1.55)	
Very high	1.41 (1.28–1.56)	
Income quartile		0.039
Very Low	Referent	
Low	1.06 (0.96–1.17)	
Intermediate	1.15 (1.04–1.27)	
High	1.15 (1.03–1.27)	
Very high	1.13 (1.02–1.26)	

Reprinted with permission of Elsevier Publishers from Abouassaly et al. (2011)
*C-statistic = 0.66, Hosmer–Lemeshow $p = 0.044$
[†]C-Statistic = 0.65, Hosmer–Lemeshow $p = 0.73$

effect on the risk of complications. If it does, then we would want to know which categories of that factor are "significant." Each category having a coefficient associated with it is being compared to the reference group (labeled "Referent" in the table) for the dummy variables representing that factor. All effects are being reported as odds ratios (OR), with 95 % confidence intervals for the odds ratios in parentheses.

For example, being 80 or older is associated with odds of complications that are 1.74 times higher than for those who are under 50 (the reference group), controlling for the other factors in the model. Or, those 80 or older have 74 % greater odds of complications compared to those under 50. Those having a Charlson score of 3 or greater have 6.22 times greater odds of developing complications, compared to those with a Charlson score of zero, and so forth. Whether each of these comparisons of a category of a factor with the reference group for that factor is significant can be discerned from the confidence interval for its odds ratio. If that confidence interval does not contain 1.0, then that odds ratio is significant. Returning to our two examples, we see that the confidence interval for the OR for age 80 or greater is 1.52–1.98. This interval does not contain 1.0, so it is significant. This means that the odds of complications for those aged 80 or over are significantly greater than for those aged less than 50. Or, the confidence interval for the OR for a Charlson score of 3 or greater is 5.18–7.48. Again, this interval does not contain 1.0, so this OR is significant. Those with a Charlson score of 3 or greater have significantly greater odds of complications, compared to those with a Charlson score of zero. What do we do if we want to know whether those with a Charlson score of 3 or greater have greater odds of complications than those with Charlson scores of 2 (which is not the reference group)? What the analyst has to do is simply to change the reference group to those with a Charlson score of 2 and rerun the model. Then the OR for those with a Charlson score of 3 or greater will be with reference to those with a Charlson score of 2. This latter comparison may or may not be of interest. We see that several of the ORs are not significant, because their CIs do contain 1.0: the ORs for fiscal years 2000–2005, the OR for the intermediate hospital-volume quartile, and the OR for the low income quintile fall into this category.

Measures of empirical consistency and discriminatory power are reported at the end of the table. The starred (*) entries are for radical nephrectomy (the other two entries are for partial nephrectomy, whose results are not shown). We see that the AUC ("C-statistic") is only 0.66. This is not considered acceptable discriminatory power for a logistic regression model. We notice, too, that the p value for the Hosmer–Lemeshow chi-squared is just significant, at $p = 0.044$. This also suggests a model that does not have a particularly good fit to the data. That very significant explanatory variable effects can coexist with a marginally performing model here is due to the very large sample size. In this case, there is a considerable amount of power for detecting "significant" effects, even though model performance is less than impressive on the whole.

Caffeine, Smoking, and Parkinson Disease

Coffee drinking and cigarette smoking have both been shown, in a number of studies, to be associated with a lower risk of developing Parkinson disease, or PD (Liu et al. 2012). The authors explain the connection of Parkinson's with caffeine (p. 1200): "It has been hypothesized that caffeine and its major metabolites may protect dopaminergic neurons by antagonizing adenosine A2A receptor." With this in mind, Liu and colleagues undertook an evaluation of the influence of caffeine intake and smoking on the development of PD in a large cohort of men and women. They utilized data from the NIH-AARP Diet and Health Study on AARP members aged 50–71 from six US states and two metropolitan areas. A baseline survey on diet and lifestyle, including coffee and cigarette consumption, was answered in 1995–1996. Then a follow-up survey was conducted in 2004–2006 among surviving participants to ascertain the occurrence of major chronic diseases such as Parkinson's. After excluding cases with missing data, the sample size was 304,980 participants, 1,100 of whom had been diagnosed with PD during or after the year 2000. Caffeine intake was assessed at least 4 years before PD diagnosis for these individuals. In studies without random assignment to levels of the explanatory variables, an important means of control to ensure causal priority is to exclude certain cases. The authors explain (p. 1201): "Because caffeine intake was assessed in 1995–1996 and we were concerned that PD patients might have altered their coffee consumption, even prior to PD diagnosis, we excluded 1,094 potential cases diagnosed before 2000 from the analyses." That is, for individuals diagnosed too close to baseline (1995–1996), at which coffee consumption was measured, developing PD might actually have caused an increase in their coffee consumption. Since coffee consumption is presumed to be a cause of level of risk for PD, these patients demonstrating reverse causation had to be excluded from the study. The statistical analysis consisted of a logistic regression of PD (coded 1 if the respondent had PD, 0 otherwise) on caffeine intake plus control variables.

Participants with higher caffeine intake were more likely to be male, Caucasian, and less physically active. Caffeine intake was strongly associated with cigarette smoking. Higher coffee consumption was associated with a lower risk for PD. But once cigarette smoking was controlled in the analysis, this effect only held for caffeinated coffee. Moreover, consumption of other caffeinated beverages (e.g., tea, soft drinks) was not related to the risk of PD (Liu et al. 2012). The principal findings are explained by the authors (p. 1204) and shown in Fig. 7.4:

> Duration of smoking was strongly associated with lower PD risk; further adjustment for caffeine intake barely changed the risk estimates for smoking (Web Table 3). Joint analysis of smoking duration and caffeine intake showed that smoking was associated with lower PD risk within each level of caffeine intake (Figure 1; for all subgroups, Ptrend ≤ 0.01). In contrast, higher caffeine intake was significantly associated with lower PD risk among never smokers (Ptrend $= 0.04$), but the monotonic trend was less clear among ever smokers. Nevertheless, compared with never smokers with low caffeine intake, long-term smokers with high caffeine intake had the lowest risk of PD. The statistical test for a potential interaction between smoking and caffeine intake was far from statistically significant ($P = 0.57$).

As the authors made clear, there is no interaction between smoking and caffeine intake in their effects on the probability of developing PD. The effects of caffeine intake and smoking appear to be cumulative in reducing the risk for PD, with the lowest odds of developing PD shown by the group with the last bar on the right in the figure. This is the group with high caffeine intake who are either past smokers who smoked for 30 or more years or who are current smokers. Their odds ratio of 0.48 is comparing their odds of PD to those on the far left (with an OR = 1.00), the reference category. Thus, the lowest risk group for PD has odds of developing PD that are only about half (i.e., 0.48) the odds of those with low caffeine intake who never smoked. Controlling for age at baseline, race, physical activity, and gender do not alter these findings.

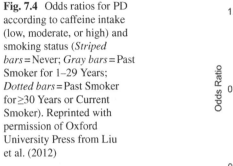

Fig. 7.4 Odds ratios for PD according to caffeine intake (low, moderate, or high) and smoking status (*Striped bars* = Never; *Gray bars* = Past Smoker for 1–29 Years; *Dotted bars* = Past Smoker for ≥30 Years or Current Smoker). Reprinted with permission of Oxford University Press from Liu et al. (2012)

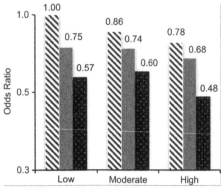

PSA as a Predictor of Prostate Cancer

Crawford and colleagues (2011) conducted a nonexperimental study to determine the prognostic value of initial PSA levels in men for identifying the risk of developing prostate cancer (PC). Their contention is that men with a *first* PSA reading between 1.5 and 4.0 face the same future risk of PC as those with a PSA level above 4.0 in any given examination (Crawford et al. 2011). Their database consisted of men in the Health Alliance Plan of Henry Ford Health System between 1997 and 2008. They were at least 40 years old, had initial PSA values between 0 and 4.0 ng/mL, and had a minimum of 4 years of follow-up after their first PSA. As in the previous study, exclusionary criteria were employed to exercise control over direction of causality (p. 1744):

> To assess the future predictive value of a first PSA test, patients could not have been in the system for less than 6 months (to rule out the possibility of referral for prostate cancer) and patients could not have received a diagnosis of prostate cancer within 6 months of baseline PSA (otherwise, possibly representing the PSA that initiated biopsy and diagnosis). These exclusionary criteria were designed to ensure temporal separation between the baseline PSA and a subsequent diagnosis of cancer.

The study endpoint was a diagnosis of PC, coded 1 for such a diagnosis, and 0 otherwise. This was then analyzed via logistic regression using initial PSA value as the primary predictor. Initial PSA value was dichotomized as <1.5 vs. 1.5–4. The authors' description of their analytic technique is instructive (p. 1744):

> Multivariate analysis, adjusting for age and race, was performed using SAS v9.1.3. Initially, the relative risk of prostate cancer was determined for all subjects based on a PSA threshold of 1.5 ng/mL. The PSA threshold analysis was subsequently stratified by race, controlling for age. To determine optimal PSA threshold, receiver operating characteristic curves were constructed and then the sums of sensitivity and specificity were evaluated. Area under the receiver operating characteristic curve (AUC) was used to determine the predictive ability of PSA values for prostate cancer. A perfect test has an AUC of 1.0, whereas a test with no diagnostic value has an AUC < 0.5.

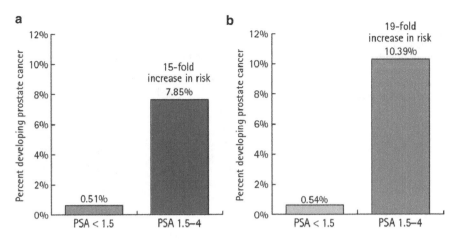

Fig. 7.5 Risks of prostate cancer for the entire sample (**a**) and African-Americans Only (**b**). Reprinted with permission of John Wiley and Sons, publishers, from Crawford et al. (2011)

We notice that the authors mention the statistical software package they used to analyze the data as being SAS v 9.1.3. SAS output has been shown in previous chapters. We see, also, that some analyses were "stratified" by race, that is, analyses were run separately for different racial groups, and included age as a control variable. Apparently the authors explored different PSA cutoffs for the dichotomized PSA explanatory variable but found that 1.5 provided the greatest AUC and the best values of sensitivity and specificity. Moreover, AUC was used to assess discriminatory power of the model, as has been illustrated above for the GSS example.

The primary study findings are illustrated in Fig. 7.5.

As illustrated in the figure, and emphasized by the authors, men with a baseline PSA ≥ 1.5 ng/mL had odds of prostate cancer that were 15 times higher than those with PSA < 1.5 ng/mL. For African-American men, those with PSA ≥ 1.5 ng/mL had a PC risk that was 19 times higher than those with PSA < 1.5 ng/mL. How good was the researchers' logistic regression model for forecasting PC? The AUC results are depicted in Fig. 7.6.

The figure shows that the AUC was 0.873, which suggests excellent discriminatory power for the authors' model. Sensitivity and specificity, according to the figure, are both about 0.80.

Vitamin D Deficiency and Frailty

Another study employing logistic regression and reporting the AUC for the model is by Wilhelm-Leen et al (2010). Their primary study endpoint was frailty in older persons, described as a "multidimensional phenotype that describes declining physical function and a vulnerability to adverse health outcomes in the setting of

Fig. 7.6 Receiver operating
characteristic curve for PC
prediction for all study
patients. Reprinted with
permission of John Wiley and
Sons, publishers, from
Crawford et al. (2011)

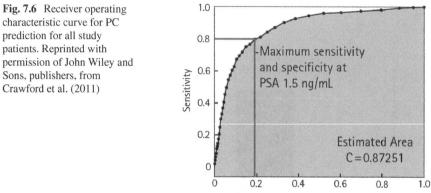

physical stress such as illness or hospitalization" (Wilhelm-Leen et al., p. 171). Their hypothesis was that 25-hydroxyvitamin D deficiency would be predictive of frailty in older adults, controlling for advanced age and chronic medical conditions. They utilized data from the Third National Health and Nutrition Evaluation Survey, a nationally representative survey of the health status of persons residing in the USA collected in the period 1988–1994. Their sample consisted of 5.048 persons aged 60 or older with 25-hydroxyvitamin D data available. Frailty was coded as 1 for frail, 0 for not frail. This was based on respondents having three or more of the following conditions: low body weight for height, slow walking, weakness, exhaustion, and low physical activity. The authors controlled for several factors in their analysis, such as age, sex, and, poverty status, and various comorbidities, such as diabetes, chronic lung disease, and chronic kidney disease. The logistic regression results for Whites are shown in Table 7.7.

In the original table title (not reproduced here), AUC was reported as 0.767. This indicates a model with acceptable discriminatory power. We see, also, that the primary explanatory variable, vitamin D, has the expected effect. Those with D level less than 15 ng mL^{-1} have an estimated odds of being frail that is over three times greater (3.7, to be exact) than those with D levels greater than or equal to 30 ng mL^{-1}. And this holds while controlling for age, gender, poverty-to-income ratio (PIR), and various comorbidities. As for the other factors, there appears to be no significant gender difference in the risk of frailty. But not surprisingly, the probability of being frail increases with age, a lower PIR, and the conditions of arthritis, nonskin cancer, chronic kidney disease, cardiovascular disease, and diabetes.

Heat Sensitivity in MS Patients

Sensitivity to environmental heat is a well-known concomitant of multiple sclerosis (MS) that exacerbates MS symptoms. Flensner et al. (2011) examined the effects of

Table 7.7 Logistic regression results for frailty of white respondents

	OR	95 % CI
Vitamin D (ng mL⁻¹)		
≥30	Reference	–
15–<30	1.0	0.6–1.7
<15	3.7	2.1–6.8
Age (years)		
60–69	Reference	–
70–79	1.9	1.3–2.8
≥80	2.5	1.4–4.5
Sex		
Male	Reference	–
Female	1.2	0.8–1.8
Poverty to income ratio (PIR)		
PIR≥2	Reference	–
PIR<2	1.9	1.3–2.6
Comorbidity		
Arthritis	3.8	2.2–6.5
Cancer, nonskin	1.9	1.2–2.9
Chronic liver disease	1.4	0.7–2.7
Chronic lung disease	1.4	0.8–2.3
Chronic kidney disease	1.7	1.1–2.6
Cardiovascular disease	1.8	1.2–2.6
Diabetes	1.6	1.1–2.3

Reprinted with permission of John Wiley and Sons, publishers, from Wilhelm-Leen et al. (2010)

heat sensitivity on a variety of common MS symptoms. Their data were drawn from 334 MS sufferers in the Swedish MS Register. Inclusion criteria were being diagnosed with MS, having an Expanded Disability Status Score (EDSS) between 0 and 6.5, and being between 20 and 65 years of age (Flensner et al. 2011). Information was gathered from respondents via mailed questionnaires. Heat sensitivity was based on a single question: "Are you sensitive to heat?" (Flensner et al. (2011), p. 2). This was coded simply "yes" (1) and "no" (0). Table 7.8 presents logistic regression results for the effects of heat sensitivity and the EDSS score on several MS symptoms. The authors' table title notes that each symptom is coded "1 = never to sometimes, 2 = usually to always." We should note that, although the study endpoint for logistic regression is usually coded 1 and 0, this coding is not a requirement. Any two numerical codes will suffice, provided they are recognized by the software used to analyze the data.

As is evident, heat sensitivity has significant effects on six of the eight symptoms shown. In all cases, heat sensitivity exacerbates the symptom. For example, those who are heat sensitive have odds of fatigue that are about two-and-a-half times greater than those who are not heat sensitive. Similar effects are seen for leg weakness, concentration difficulties, pain, paraesthesia, and urination urgency. EDSS is also associated with several symptoms. Unique to this analysis is the reporting of a

Table 7.8 Logistic regression analysis of common MS symptoms on EDSS score and heat sensitivity

MS symptoms	EDSS			Heat sensitivity			
	OR	95 % CI	P-value	OR	95 % CI	P-value	R^2 Nagelkerke
Fatigue	1.15	0.98–1.32	0.086	2.55	1.48–4.25	<0.001	0.136
Leg weakness	1.51	1.26–1.81	<0.001	2.21	1.24–3.93	0.007	0.274
Spasms	1.79	1.43–2.22	<0.001	1.65	0.77–350	0.194	0.232
Balance problems	1.62	1.34–1.94	<0.001	1.48	0.83–2.65	0.181	0.285
Concentration difficulties	1.08	0.92–1.28	0.354	3.40	1.85–6.25	<0.001	0.123
Pain	1.09	0.92–1.29	0.344	3.55	1.87–6.77	<0.001	0.136
Paraesthesia	1.20	1.02–1.41	0.026	2.10	1.21–3.64	0.008	0.095
Urination urgency	1.27	1.05–1.54	0.016	2.75	1.28–5.90	0.009	0.256

Reprinted from Flensner et al. (2011), an open-access journal

pseudo-R^2 value: "R^2 Nagelkerke." For each MS symptom, R^2 pertains to the logistic regression model containing two predictors: EDSS and heat sensitivity. The Nagelkerke R^2 is similar to Pseudo R_2^2 in Table 7.1 and discussed above. It is a good estimate of the quantitative variable that underlies a binary indicator. In this case, in which the study endpoints refer to the frequency or intensity of MS symptoms, such a quantitative underlying variable is quite plausible. The advantage to the Nagelkerke R^2 is that it is frequently reported as a standard part of logistic regression software. The disadvantage is that, unlike the linear regression R^2, Pseudo R_1^2, and Pseudo R_2^2, it does not have an explained-variance interpretation (DeMaris 2002). It simply indicates the degree of discriminatory power of the model, on a scale from 0 to 1. Apparently, the model demonstrates the greatest predictive efficacy for the study endpoint "balance problems."

This chapter has dealt primarily with binary logistic regression, a technique that is appropriate whenever we have a dichotomous outcome variable. But what should we do if we have a dichotomous outcome but it represents an event that occurs to cases that are followed longitudinally? For example, we might follow patients from the time of their diagnosis with a potentially fatal disease to see what factors affect whether they die. It turns out that we do not just want to perform a logistic regression with death as the binary outcome as our analytic strategy. The reason is that we want to take account of *how long they survive until death*, not just whether they die or not. There will also be patients who are still alive at the end of the observation period. These patients have survival times that are said to be "censored." Rather than just treat these cases as though they are "safe," we incorporate the censoring into the analyses. These nuances of time-to-event data are all readily incorporated into the technique called *survival analysis*, the subject of the next chapter.

Chapter 8
Survival Analysis

This chapter takes up the topic of *survival analysis*, one of the most frequently employed statistical techniques in medical research. This is the statistical tool we use when we follow cases over time to see whether they experience a particular event. Because the event in question is often death, the period of time from inception of risk for the event until the occurrence of the event has come to be called *survival time*. And the technique has come to be known as survival analysis. However, in fields other than medicine it is also referred to as *failure-time analysis, reliability analysis, duration analysis,* or *event history analysis* (Allison 2010). The event in question need not just be death. In fact, any time we are interested in studying the length of time until occurrence of an event and how characteristics of cases affect that time, survival analysis is relevant. The event in question could be the development of prostate cancer (Pettaway et al. 2011), recurrence of prostate cancer after radical prostatectomy (O'Brien et al. 2010), the occurrence of heart failure (Khawaja et al. 2012), death within 90 days of radical cystectomy (Morgan et al. 2011), the development of incident dementia (Lieb et al. 2009), and so on.

Why Special Methods Are Required

Why are special methods required for the study of survival time? Suppose that we randomly assigned men between the ages of 40 and 50 to be treated with either dutasteride (trade name: Avodart) or a placebo and then follow them for the next 10 years with digital rectal exams and PSA measurements every 6 months to see if there is any difference between groups in the rate of development of prostate cancer (PC; established via prostate biopsy). For these men we have baseline (e.g., pre-treatment) measures of educational level, marital status, and other demographics. We also take measures at each 6-month follow-up visit of nutritional intake, smoking status, BMI, and other lifestyle habits. These latter are explanatory variables

A. DeMaris and S.H. Selman, *Converting Data into Evidence: A Statistics Primer for the Medical Practitioner*, DOI 10.1007/978-1-4614-7792-1_8,
© Springer Science+Business Media New York 2013

whose values can change over time and are referred to as *time-varying covariates*. A simplistic statistical approach here might be just to create a binary variable, Y, coded 1 for whether the subject developed PC at any time over the 10-year period and 0 otherwise, and then estimate a logistic regression for the log-odds of developing cancer as a function of treatment status and other study covariates. However, this would be wasteful of important information. First, it makes a difference whether a unit develops PC early in the study as opposed to toward the end of the study. The simplistic approach ignores the *timing* of occurrence of the event of interest. In fact, this timing is a key endpoint for the study. Second, those at the end of the study who haven't yet developed PC are being treated as though they are "safe" from the event. But they may develop PC after the study is over; it's just that we aren't able to observe their total survival time in the noncancer state. These units are said to have their survival time *censored* (by the end of the study) and are therefore referred to as *censored cases*.

An alternative approach might be to use survival time in the noncancer state as the study endpoint. Then we could just do a linear regression of survival time on treatment status plus study covariates. This is also problematic: how do we code survival time for censored cases? Assigning the time from beginning of the study to when they were last observed as their survival time is a poor strategy. The reason is that this value is surely an underestimate of actual survival time and will lead to biased estimates of predictor effects (Allison 2010). Also, in either the simplistic logistic regression or linear regression approaches, it is not clear how to incorporate time-varying covariates. Including in the model separate measures of each predictor for all follow-up times is not only cumbersome. It can also produce biased estimates because of causal ambiguity. For example, someone who develops PC early on may change their nutritional habits, stop smoking, and lose weight as a consequence. Hence time-varying covariates measured after the event may themselves be caused by the event and cannot plausibly be "predictors" of survival time (Allison 2010). All of these difficulties that are due to the inability of other techniques to handle censoring and time-varying covariates are easily remedied using survival-analysis methods. We now turn to those techniques.

Elemental Terms and Concepts

We begin with some definitions. The *inception of risk* is the moment at which units come under the risk for an event. The *beginning of observation* is the moment at which we begin following them in a study. In the dutasteride example, we are assuming an inception of risk of age 40–50. That is, we assume that men do not come under the risk for PC until at least age 40–50. This may not be correct, however. The risk for PC may start much earlier in life. If the risk for PC actually begins at, say, age 30, but the beginning of observation is not until age 40–50, then the sample is said to be *left-truncated*. This means that they have already been at risk for the event before they come under observation. Survival analysis is readily adapted to the problem of left truncation. The *risk set* is the collection of units at any given time who are still at risk for the event of interest. So if we start with 1,000 men, total (500 in each treatment group), then the initial risk set is 1,000. If after 5 years there have been 120 cases of PC, then the risk set at that point in time is 880 and so forth. We have already defined censoring as the incomplete observation of survival time due to the ending of observation. This is further referred to as *right censoring*. (Left censoring occurs when units have already experienced the event of interest when recruited into the study; such units are then dropped from the study.) Sometimes units drop out of the study voluntarily before the end, or they are removed from the study for other reasons, such as death due to some other cause. These units are also treated as right-censored cases in survival analysis. Finally, the two most important components in survival analysis are the survival function and the hazard function. The *survival function* is the probability of surviving (i.e., continuing along without having experienced the event of interest) to any particular point in time. It's called a "function" because it depends on time. The *hazard function* is approximately the instantaneous probability of experiencing the event for someone in the risk set at a particular moment in time. It, too, varies over time.

An Example

We draw on data presented in Hosmer and Lemeshow (1999). A large HMO wanted to evaluate the survival time of its HIV+ members using a follow-up study. One hundred subjects were enrolled in the study from January 1, 1989 to December 31, 1991. The study ended on December 31, 1995. After a confirmed diagnosis of HIV (inception of risk), members were followed until death due to AIDS or AIDS-related complications, until the end of the study, or until the subject was lost to follow-up. There were no deaths due to other causes. The study endpoint is survival time after a confirmed diagnosis of HIV. Since subjects entered the study at different times over a 3-year period, the maximum possible follow-up time is different for each study participant. Possible predictors of survival time were collected at enrollment into the study. The variables involved in the study are shown in Table 8.1.

Table 8.2 shows the data records for the first ten cases in the study.

We see that the first subject was diagnosed with HIV on 15 May of 1990 and died from AIDS on 14 October, 1990. Thus, this person only survived 5 months after diagnosis. He or she was 46 years old at diagnosis and did not have a history of IV drug use. That CENSOR = 1 tells us that this person's survival time ended in death. Subject ID 2, on the other hand, shows a survival time of 6 months from diagnosis until 20 March 1990, at which point they were lost to follow-up (CENSOR = 0). This 35-year-old did have a history of IV drug use. The longest surviving member in this group of 10 is ID 5, a 36-year-old without a history of IV drug use. This person survived 22 months until dying of AIDS.

Table 8.1 Variables in the HMO-HIV+ study

Variable	Description	Codes/units
ID	Subject ID Code	1–100
ENTDATE	Entry date	day/month/year
ENDDATE	End date	day/month/year
TIME	Survival Time	number of months between Entry date and End date
AGE	Age	age in years at enrollment
DRUG	History of IV Drug Use	0 = No 1 = Yes
CENSOR	Follow-Up Status	1 = Death due to AIDS or AIDS related factors 0 = Alive at study end or lost to follow-up

Table 8.2 Data records for the first ten cases in the HMO-HIV+ study

ID	ENTDATE	ENDDATE	TIME	AGE	DRUG	CENSOR
1	15may90	14oct90	5	46	0	1
2	19sep89	20mar90	6	35	1	0
3	21apr91	20dec91	8	30	1	1
4	03jan91	04apr91	3	30	1	1
5	18sep89	19jul91	22	36	0	1
6	18mar91	17apr91	1	32	1	0
7	11nov89	11jun90	7	36	1	1
8	25nov89	25aug90	9	31	1	1
9	11feb91	13may91	3	48	0	1
10	11aug89	11aug90	12	47	0	1

Estimating the Survival Function

It is typically of interest to estimate the survival function for individuals at risk of an event. That is, we want to see how quickly or slowly they succumb to the event of interest, in this case, death. In medicine, the most widely used method for estimating survival functions is the Kaplan–Meier (KM) estimator, also known as the *product-limit estimator*. It is a nonparametric technique because it does not rely on knowledge of the underlying distribution of survival time for the population of interest. In fact, this distribution is typically unknown, anyway. How does it work? Let's use it to calculate a few survival probabilities for the HMO-HIV+ data.

We are interested in the following: for each time at which subjects were at risk for death, we want to know the probability of surviving until that point in time. As Hosmer and Lemeshow (1999) note, survival to any point in time should be considered a series of steps. It's analogous to a toddler making his or her first steps. In order to walk five steps, the first four steps have to be made successfully. We use both the event and censoring times to determine what that "success rate" is. We begin at "time 0," the beginning of observation, which is also the inception of risk.

Since everyone is alive at that point, the survival probability for time 0 is 1.0. In our sample, 15 people died within the next month. The conditional probability of dying in the first month is therefore 15/100, or 0.15. Therefore the probability of surviving the first month at risk is $1 - 0.15 = 0.85$. Now, there are 85 people left who are still at risk of dying of aids. Two of those people are censored in the first month. So we need to reduce the risk set by two; it is now $85 - 2 = 83$. However, the survival probability remains at 0.85; it only changes when there is another death. Then five people die of AIDS in the next month, i.e., month 2 of the study. The conditional probability of dying in the second month, given survival through the first month, is then $5/83 = 0.0602$. This means that the conditional probability of surviving the second month, given that one survived the first, is $1 - 0.0602 = 0.9398$. The probability of surviving 2 months is now the probability of surviving the first month times the probability of surviving the second month, given that one survived the first. That is, the survival probability for month 2 is $0.85 \times 0.9398 = 0.7988$. At this point, there are 78 people left in the risk set. Of these, five are censored in month 2, leaving only 73 people in the risk set for month 3. By month 3, there are ten more deaths. The conditional probability of dying in the third month, given survival through the second is then $10/73 = 0.1370$. Thus, the conditional probability of surviving the third month, given that one survived the second, is $1 - 0.1370 = 0.8630$. The probability of surviving 3 months is now the probability of surviving 2 months times the probability of surviving the third, given that one survived to the second, or $0.7988 \times 0.8630 = 0.6984$. The calculations are continued in this fashion until either everybody dies, at which point the survival probability becomes zero, or the remaining cases are censored. When all that's left are censored cases, the survival probability remains constant at its last known value.

Table 8.3 presents a partial printout of the survival function based on the KM estimator for all 100 cases in the HMO-HIV+ study.

Output is from a popular statistical software package called SAS. Shown are "Survival," the survival probability for each time period, and "Failure," which is just $1 -$ Survival. This is therefore the probability of dying by each time period. For example, the probability of surviving to month 7 is 0.4701 and the probability of dying by month 7 is $1 - 0.4701 = 0.5299$. The censored observations are listed individually and starred. The last survival probability shown is 0.0389 for 58 months. Thus, there is only a 4 % chance in this sample of surviving 58 months before succumbing to AIDS. The mean survival time (not shown) is 14.59 months. But the mean is not a reliable estimator of average survival time when there are censoring times greater than the largest event time, as is the case here. A much better estimator of average survival time is the median, which is 7 months. The median is the survival time such that about half of the cases survive at least that long. Figure 8.1 shows a plot of the survival probabilities against time in the study.

This figure takes on the classic "ski-slope" shape of all survival functions. The survival curve begins at a value of 1.0 in the upper left corner of the plot. This corresponds to time 0, which is the beginning of the study. It then descends in value until the last survival probability, which in this case, is 0.0389. The censored cases are shown on the survival curve as small circles.

Table 8.3 Partial printout of survival probabilities for the HMO-HIV+ study

```
Product-Limit Survival Estimates
```

Time	Survival	Failure	Survival Standard error	Number Failed	Number Left
0.0000	1.0000	0	0	0	100
1.0000	0.8500	0.1500	0.0357	15	85
1.0000*	.	.	.	15	84
1.0000*	.	.	.	15	83
2.0000	0.7988	0.2012	0.0402	20	78
2.0000*	.	.	.	20	77
2.0000*	.	.	.	20	76
2.0000*	.	.	.	20	75
2.0000*	.	.	.	20	74
2.0000*	.	.	.	20	73
3.0000	0.6894	0.3106	0.0473	30	63
3.0000*	.	.	.	30	62
3.0000*	.	.	.	30	61
4.0000	0.6442	0.3558	0.0493	34	57
4.0000*	.	.	.	34	56
5.0000	0.5636	0.4364	0.0517	41	49
6.0000	0.5406	0.4594	0.0521	43	47
6.0000*	.	.	.	43	46
7.0000	0.4701	0.5299	0.0526	49	40
.	.	(cases omitted)			
.	.				
.	.				
54.0000	0.0778	0.9222	0.0324	78	5
56.0000*	.	.	.	78	4
57.0000	0.0584	0.9416	0.0296	79	3
58.0000	0.0389	0.9611	0.0253	80	2
60.0000*	.	.	.	80	1
60.0000*	.	.	.	80	0

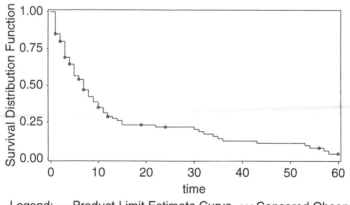

Legend: —Product-Limit Estimate Curve ∘∘∘ Censored Observations

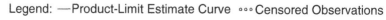

Fig. 8.1 Plot of the survival function for the HMO-HIV+ study

Comparing Survival Functions Across Groups

We might ask whether the survival experience is different for one group vs. another. For example, does it make a difference if one had a history of IV drug use? The null hypothesis is that the survivor functions are the same in the two groups. In other words, the probability distribution of survival time is exactly the same for each group, with each having the same mean survival time. Another statement of the null hypothesis is that the survival probability is exactly the same for each group at each time. The alternative hypothesis is that one group's survival probabilities are uniformly higher or lower than the other's. This is easily tested when employing the KM estimator. The most commonly used test is the *log-rank test*, although the *Wilcoxon test* is a popular alternative. Both tests compare the observed numbers of events (e.g., deaths) at each time to the expected numbers of events under the null. And both are distributed as chi-squared when the null hypothesis is true (Allison 2010). Both are also nonparametric tests. They are particularly effective when one group's survival probability is uniformly higher than the other's across all time periods. The log-rank test is more powerful at detecting differences between groups that occur at later points in time. It is also more closely related to tests for group differences that are done within the framework of Cox's proportional hazards model, which is discussed below (Allison 2010). Neither is reliable in the situation in which the groups' survival curves "cross." This would happen if one group has a higher survival probability at each time up to some specific time, after which its survival probability becomes lower than the other group's. This is not a common occurrence. A plot of survival functions in the HMO-HIV+ study for groups defined by IV drug use is shown in Fig. 8.2.

In the plot, the upper curve is for those with no IV drug use; the lower curve is for those with a history of IV drug use. It is evident that those without drug use have substantially higher survival probabilities at each time until about 55 months, at

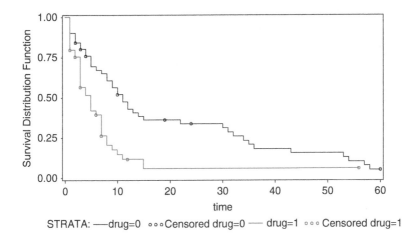

Fig. 8.2 Survivor functions for groups defined by IV drug-use status

which point both groups' survival probabilities tend to converge to a low value (about 0.04). Is this group difference in survival curves significant? The log-rank statistic is 11.86, with a p value of 0.0006, whereas the Wilcoxon statistic is 10.91, with a p value of 0.001 (results not shown). Hence, according to either test, the survival experience is significantly better for those without a history of IV drug use.

Regression Models for Survival Data

With random assignment to treatment, there may be no need to control for any other factors in examining treatment-group differences in survival. In this case, differences between survival rates according to treatment-group status can be tested using either the *log-rank* or *Wilcoxon* tests applied to survival–function estimates generated using the KM technique. On the other hand, we may want to control for other covariates, especially if the data are from an observational study, as in the HMO-HIV+ study discussed here. Although the KM technique lets us examine group differences in the survival function, it does not allow controlling for other covariates. For this purpose there are regression models for survival data.

One type of model uses logistic regression, but not in the simplistic manner described above. The approach described now is especially useful when survival time is not precisely measured. For example, in the dutasteride study described in the beginning of this section, men are followed up every 6 months. So, at best, we only know survival time in 6-month intervals, rather than the exact time from inception of risk until the occurrence of PC. One way to proceed is to create a new dataset containing a separate record for each 6-month period in which a man is cancer free. On that record we put all of his characteristics, including treatment-group status, that are of interest as predictors of PC. This includes the values of any time-varying covariates, coded according to their values in that 6-month period. For each man, there will be as many records as there are 6-month periods at which he is still at risk of developing PC. The maximum number of records a man can contribute is 20; two for each year of follow-up. Once he has developed PC or is censored due to some unforeseen exigency (e.g., lost to follow-up, dies, etc.), he no longer contributes records to the dataset. On all records for a given man who contracts PC, the study endpoint, Y, is coded 0, except for the last record, on which he's coded 1. On all records of censored cases—including those censored by the end of observation, Y is coded 0 throughout. This new dataset is said to be in *person–period format*. This terminology emphasizes that each record in the data set is a period's worth of measures contributed by a single person. We then apply ordinary logistic regression analysis to this dataset to regress Y on time period (coded using 19 dummies to represent the 20 time periods), treatment-group status, and the additional covariates. Although it seems that we are artificially inflating the sample size by converting to person–period format, it turns out that this approach is statistically sound (see, e.g., Allison 1982). This approach is referred to as a *discrete-time hazard model*.

Cox's Proportional Hazards Model

When time is more precisely measured, say in months, days, hours, etc., we want to treat it as a continuous variable, that is, a variable with a precise *continuum* of quantitative values. There are two ways to proceed. One is to use a regression model for survival time itself. The response variable in the regression is actually the log of time. This ensures that the estimated survival time is always a positive quantity. This type of model is called an *accelerated failure-time* (AFT) *model* and is estimated using the technique of maximum likelihood. The drawback to it is that we must know, ahead of time, what the probability distribution of survival time is. This distribution determines both the survival and hazard functions. (Recall that the hazard function refers to the way in which the hazard of event occurrence varies over time.) If the wrong probability distribution is used, then model estimates of both the effect coefficients and their standard errors could be biased (this is bad).

Back in the 1970s the British statistician Sir David Cox came up with a unique solution to this dilemma. He partitioned the likelihood function for AFT models into two parts. He noticed that one part was only a function of the regression coefficients, while the other was a function of both the regression coefficients and the hazard function. So he discarded the second part of the likelihood function and only used the first part to find the regression coefficients that maximized it. The technique is called *partial likelihood* estimation, and the resulting model is known either as the *Cox regression model* or the *proportional hazards model* (Allison 2010; DeMaris 2004; Hosmer and Lemeshow 1999). The beauty of this approach is that the underlying distribution of survival time is immaterial: we simply ignore how the hazard varies with time and focus on how explanatory variables affect the hazard. The response variable in the model is the log of the hazard rate, rather than the log of survival time. These two quantities are inversely related: the greater the hazard of the event at any given time, the shorter the survival time, and vice versa. The model easily incorporates time-varying covariates and censoring of survival times. With $\log(h_t)$ as the log of the hazard (which varies over time, represented by the subscript "t") and X_t as a time-varying covariate, the model with just two predictors (for simplicity) takes the form

$$\log(h_t) = b_1 X_t + b_2 Z.$$

The "t" subscript on X means that the values of X can change over time. On the other hand, Z is a time-invariant factor, like gender or race, that stays the same over time. Notice that there is no intercept in the model. This is part of the information that's discarded in the likelihood function. The interpretation of the coefficients is very similar to interpretation of coefficients in logistic regression. Exponentiating a coefficient gives us the equivalent of an odds ratio, except that it's called a *hazard ratio* in this model. For example, $\exp(b_1)$ is the multiplicative factor by which the hazard of the event increases (or decreases) for each unit increase in X_t, controlling for Z. A similar interpretation applies to b_2.

The Cox model is not as efficient as the AFT model, because it discards some information in the likelihood function. "Inefficiency" refers to the Cox coefficients having larger standard errors than in the AFT model, which means the Cox model isn't as powerful as the AFT model. However, Cox regression more than makes up for this loss of efficiency by its robustness: the Cox model gives good results regardless of the underlying probability distribution of survival time. The same can't be said for the AFT. The one limitation, of course, is that the Cox model doesn't allow us to examine how the hazard rate varies over time. Nevertheless, it does allow estimation of the survival function and the manner in which the survival probability depends on the explanatory variables in the model. Because of its positive features, the Cox model is perhaps the most widely used regression model in survival analysis.

Modeling the Hazard of Death Due to AIDS

Table 8.4 presents the results of a Cox regression for the hazard of death due to AIDS for the 100 subjects in the HMO-HIV+ study. The two explanatory variables are the subject's age and history of IV drug use. Recall that the latter is coded as a dummy variable with 1 representing "used drugs" and 0 representing "did not use drugs."

The first number of importance, highlighted in bold, is the likelihood-ratio chi-squared test. This is analogous to the F test in linear regression or the model chi-squared test in logistic regression. It's a test for whether the model as a whole is "significant." That is, the null hypothesis for this test is that both population coefficients corresponding to age and drug use equal zero. As is evident, this hypothesis is resoundingly rejected at $p < 0.0001$. Regression coefficients for the variables "age" and "drug" (use) are listed under "Parameter Estimate." We see that both age and drug use are significant predictors of death. The older the subject is, the greater the hazard of death at any given time. Exponentiating the age coefficient of 0.09151 provides the hazard ratio of 1.096 that is shown at the far right. This is interpreted thus: each year older the subject is at the beginning of observation raises the hazard of death due to AIDS by a factor of 1.096, or about 9.6 %. Similarly, the hazard ratio for drug use is 2.563. This means that the hazard of death at any time is 2.563 times greater for those who used drugs than for those who didn't.

Table 8.4 Cox regression results for the HMO-HIV+ study

Testing Global Null Hypothesis: BETA=0				
Test	Chi-Square	DF	Pr > ChiSq	
Likelihood Ratio	**34.9819**	2	<0.0001	
Analysis of Maximum Likelihood Estimates				
Variable	DF	Parameter Estimate	Standard Error	Chi-Square	Pr > ChiSq	Hazard Ratio
age	1	0.09151	0.01849	24.5009	<0.0001	1.096
drug	1	0.94108	0.25550	13.5662	0.0002	2.563

Predictive Efficacy of the Cox Model

How do we measure the predictive efficacy or discriminatory power of the Cox model? R^2 values are not typically reported in hazard modeling because there is no commonly accepted analog of the R^2 in linear regression. Instead, medical researchers are coming to rely more and more on an analog of the AUC in logistic regression. The measure in question is called the *concordance index* (or *c* index) and is described by Harrell et al. (1996) in their influential article. Here is how it is calculated. We consider *all possible pairs of patients*, at least one of whom has "died," i.e., experienced the event of interest. That means that if there were, e.g., 10 patients, 2 of whom had died, we would compare 16 pairs of patients: each of the eight surviving patients would be paired with each of the two deceased patients. We then generate a predicted survival time for each patient in the study based on the Cox regression results. If the predicted survival time is larger for the patient who lived longer, the predictions for that pair are determined to be concordant with the actual outcomes. Or, if one patient died and the other is known to have survived at least to the survival time of the first, the second patient is assumed to have outlived the first, and this is also a concordant pair. On the other hand, a patient pair is unusable if both patients died at the same time, or if one died and the other is still alive but hasn't been followed long enough to tell whether he or she will outlive the deceased one. The *c* index is defined by the authors as "the proportion of all usable patient pairs in which the predictions and outcomes are concordant" (Harrell et al. 1996, p. 370). As with the AUC, a value of 0.5 means the Cox model has no discriminatory power, and a value of 1.0 indicates perfect discriminatory power. Similar guidelines obtain for the *c* index as for the AUC: values above 0.7 indicate acceptable discriminatory power, values above 0.8 indicate excellent discriminatory power, and values above 0.9 indicate outstanding discriminatory power. Unfortunately, the *c* index is not available in all Cox regression software. For example, it is not part of SAS version 9.1, which we used to analyze the HMO-HIV+ data above. Therefore we are not able to report it for that analysis. But we will see it used in the applications to be discussed next.

Applications: Survival Analysis in Action

Predicting 90-Day Survival After Radical Cystectomy

Our first application of the Cox model is from a study by Morgan and colleagues (2011) on the risk of mortality of bladder cancer patients within 90 days following radical cystectomy (RC). The authors' study is motivated by their observation that among those 75 years old or more, bladder cancer is the fifth leading cancer diagnosis. Moreover, they argue that it is not always clear whether RC is safe and efficacious for this particular patient population (Morgan et al. 2011). The purpose of the authors' study is to develop a *predictive nomogram* to augment clinical decisions regarding a patient's suitability for RC. A nomogram is a mathematical formula based on statistical analysis of patient outcomes. It is designed so that points can be assigned for various patient characteristics. The point total is then translated into a probability of surviving a particular procedure. As the authors note (p. 830): "Particularly, individualized modeling in the form of multivariate nomograms benefits clinical decision making for prostate cancer and aids in outcome prediction after RC."

The study in question was a retrospective cohort study of 220 consecutive patients aged 75 or older who underwent RC for urothelial carcinoma of the bladder at Vanderbilt University Medical Center (VUMC) between 2000 and 2008. Due to missing data on key factors, 51 patients were excluded from the study, leaving 169 patients for statistical analysis. Here is the authors' description of their statistical methodology (p. 830):

> Patient information, including age, sex, race, preoperative albumin, CCI, clinical stage, pathological stage and urinary diversion type were obtained from patient charts. Preoperative serum albumin was determined close to the time of surgery and patients received no specific therapy based on serum albumin levels. Vital status was ascertained through the VUMC cancer registry, the Social Security Death Index and patient charts. Patients were censored at the date of last followup or death up to August 1, 2009. The primary study end point was 90-day mortality. Cox univariate and multivariate regression was performed to determine predictors of 90-day mortality. HRs are presented with the 95% CI. Kaplan-Meier survival curves were generated to compare unadjusted 90-day mortality by patient age and preoperative albumin. Multivariate Cox regression coefficients were used to generate the prognostic nomogram and the c-index was assessed as a measure of model accuracy.

Some commentary is in order. "HRs" are hazard ratios and they are presented along with 95 % confidence intervals (CIs). Kaplan–Meier curves are examined (but not shown here) to take an initial look at how survival probability differs according to patient age and preoperative albumin. The primary study endpoint bears comment. Normally the event of interest in survival analysis would be death, per se. However, the authors use death *within 90 days of surgery* as the event of interest. Patients with this brief a survival time after surgery would presumably not be good surgery candidates. Hence, patients in this study would be considered censored if they are still alive after 90 days postsurgery. They would also be censored if they were lost to follow-up before the end of the 90-day observation window. Although the authors also describe patients as "censored" at the date of death, this terminology is not correct. Patients who experience the event of interest—in this case, death within 90 days post-op—are not censored, since their survival time is known exactly. In fact, in survival-analysis lingo they are known as *uncensored cases*. The "multivariate Cox regression" model was used to generate the predictive nomogram. Notice also mention of the use of the c-index to assess model "accuracy," i.e., predictive efficacy.

In the following passage, the authors detail the sample distribution on the event of interest (death within 90 days of surgery) and on the characteristics of patients excluded from the study (p. 830):

> Of the 220 patients in the complete cohort 28 (12.7%) and 18 of the 169 (10.7%) in the analytical cohort died within 90 days of surgery. The 51 patients who were excluded from the analytical cohort due to incomplete preoperative information did not differ statistically

Table 8.5 Cox regression analyses predicting the hazard of mortality within 90 days [Reprinted with permission of Elsevier Publishers from Morgan et al. (2011)]

	HR (95 % CI)	p Value
Univariate		
Age (IQR 76.9, 81.8)	2.15 (1.41–3.29)	<0.001
Charlson comorbidity index (range 0–3)	1.47 (0.77–2.83)	0.25
Muscle-invasive clinical stage	1.48 (0.63–3.54)	0.37
Preop albumin (IQR 4.4, 3.7)	2.17 (1.33–3.57)	0.002
Multivariate		
Age (IQR 76.9, 81.8)	2.30 (1.22–4.32)	0.010
Charlson comorbidity index (range 0–3)	1.30 (0.53–3.18)	0.56
Muscle-invasive clinical stage	1.55 (0.55–4.34)	0.41
Preop albumin (IQR 4.4, 3.7)	2.50 (1.40–4.45)	0.002

from the final cohort in age, race, or clinical or pathological stage. However, excluded patients were more likely to undergo continent urinary diversion (18% vs. 7%, p = 0.016). Ten excluded patients (19%) died within 90 days, which was not statistically different from the rate in the analytical cohort (log rank test p = 0.14).

We see that patients were more likely to be excluded due to missing data when they underwent continent urinary diversion. Notice the use of the log rank test to test whether the death rate among the 51 excluded patients (based on KM estimation) was different from that of the analytical cohort (i.e., the 169 patients actually used in the Cox model). It was not, suggesting that the analysis was likely not biased by the exclusion of these patients. Somewhat troubling (from a statistical viewpoint, that is) is that only 18 of the 169 patients in the Cox regression experienced the event of interest. This is a fairly small subset of the data, and it is not clear how robust the findings are when so few units are in the category of interest (i.e., dead within 90 days).

Table 8.5 shows the results of the Cox regressions.

The "Univariate" results are the results of a Cox regression of the log hazard of 90-day mortality on each independent variable, one at a time. The "Multivariate" results are the result of a Cox regression of the log hazard of mortality on all four variables together. It's clear that the univariate and multivariate results are pretty much in agreement. Only two of the four factors examined here have significant effects on the risk of mortality within 90 days in either the univariate or multivariate models: age and preoperative albumin level. The effects of both age and albumin level actually get a little stronger in the multivariate results. That is, each becomes a stronger predictor of the risk of mortality when controlling for the other (along with the other two factors). The "HR" column shows hazard ratios for each effect, along with their 95 % confidence intervals. Hence, each additional year of age raises the hazard of death by a factor of 2.3, while each additional unit increase of albumin raises the hazard by a factor of 2.5. ("IQR" as shown for Age and Preop albumin refers to the interquartile range or the range of the middle half of the values for the variable. Thus, 25 % of the patients are younger than 76.9 and 25 % are older than 81.8, and so forth.) The c index for this model was 0.75 (Morgan et al. 2011), which indicates a model with acceptable predictive power.

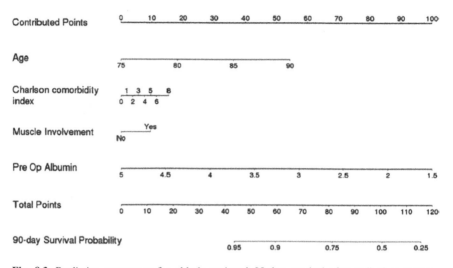

Fig. 8.3 Predictive nomogram for elderly patients' 90-day survival after radical cystectomy [Reprinted with permission of Elsevier Publishers from Morgan et al. (2011)]

Finally, Fig. 8.3 shows the predictive nomogram that can be used to estimate the 90-day survival probability for any given patient.

The idea is to choose a patient profile in terms of the attributes of age, Charlson index, muscle involvement, and pre-op albumin. For example, the legend at the bottom (not shown here) shows how to predict survival probability for an 83-year-old with muscle invasive cancer, Charlson index of 2, and pre-op albumin of 2.9. These values are located on their respective scales and then linked to their corresponding "contributed points" on the scale at the top. Then all the contributed points are summed for a total score. When doing this by inspection, we get 25 points for age, 5 points for the Charlson index, 10 points for muscle involvement, and 60 points for albumin level, for a total of 100 points. Then linking the point total with the 90-day survival probability scale just below it, we see that this patient's 90-day survival probability is 0.50. That is, he or she has a 50 % chance of surviving at least 90 days after surgery, according to the nomogram (which is based on the multivariate Cox model in Table 8.5).

Predicting Biochemical Recurrence After Radical Prostatectomy

Another example of the development of a predictive nomogram is offered by O'Brien and her colleagues (2010) in their study of biochemical recurrence (BCR) after radical prostatectomy (RP). Here is the authors' introductory statement (p. 390):

> The accurate prediction of cancer cure after radical prostatectomy (RP) allows appropriate patient counselling and enables planning of secondary treatment. Nomograms are based on mathematical formulas that consider individual patient clinicopathological details, and are proven to give more accurate predictions than those based on clinical judgment or classification of patients into risk groups [1,2]. One of the most widely used post-RP prognostic

Table 8.6 Development of the final cox model for predicting BCR after RP [Reprinted with permission of John Wiley and Sons, Publishers, from O'Brien et al. (2010)]

	Base model		Model 5		Final model	
	$N = 1{,}939$		$N = 1{,}939$		$N = 1{,}939$	
	Hazard ratio	p	Hazard ratio	p	Hazard ratio	p
Covariates						
PSA	1.05	<0.001	1.05	<0.001	1.05	<0.001
Prostate weight	0.99	0.01	0.99	0.017	0.99	0.015
% 4/5	1.02	<0.001	1.03	<0.001	1.03	<0.001
IDCP	1.74	<0.001	1.71	<0.001	1.72	<0.001
SVI	1.94	<0.001	2.08	<0.001	1.98	<0.001
ECE	1.26	0.12	1.29	0.08	0.58	0.145
PSM	2.93	<0.001	8.7	<0.001	8.58	<0.001
% 4/5 × PSM	N/A	N/A	0.98	<0.001	0.98	<0.001
% 4/5 × ECE	N/A	N/A	N/A	N/A	1.012	0.016
p (LR test)	N/A		<0.0001*		0.016†	
c Index for model	0.819		0.824		0.828	
Bootstrap c index‡					0.828	
(95 % CI)					(0.803–0.852)	

tools is the Kattan nomogram, which was first published in 1999 then revised in 2005 and 2009 [3–5]. This series of nomograms has established the importance of clinicopathological variables such as preoperative serum PSA level, Gleason grade, extracapsular extension (ECE), seminal vesicle invasion (SVI), positive surgical margins (PSM) and pelvic lymph node involvement (LNI) for predicting the risk of biochemical recurrence (BCR) after RP.

The authors' intention was to validate the Kattan nomogram with a new patient sample, and, in the process, to add some new predictive variables. These include percent of cancer with Gleason patterns 4 and/or 5 (% 4/5), prostate weight, presence or absence of intraductal carcinoma (IDCP), and tumor volume (O'Brien et al. 2010).

The sample consisted of all 2,385 consecutive RP cases processed at an Australian University Hospital between 1998 and 2007. After dropping patients based on various exclusion criteria and further eliminating those with missing data, a total of 1,939 patients were available for analysis. The study endpoint was BCR, defined as (p. 390) "a rising postoperative serum PSA of ≥0.2 ng/mL." Survival time was calculated as the time from RP to the occurrence of BCR for noncensored cases, or to the end of the study for censored cases. Cox regression was employed as the modeling technique. Once again, the authors used the c index to assess model discriminatory power (O'Brien et al. 2010). In this analysis, however, there were significant interaction effects that were incorporated into the model and resulting nomogram. In particular, % 4/5 interacted with extracapsular extension (ECE) and with positive surgical margins (PSM) in their effects on the risk for BCR. Their Cox regression results are shown in Table 8.6.

In this table we see a sequence of models: Base model, Model 5, Final model. Each successive model adds an interaction term and tests its significance. Hence, the final model contains two interaction terms: % 4/5 × PSM and % 4/5 × ECE, both of which are significant after controlling for all other factors in the model. In the

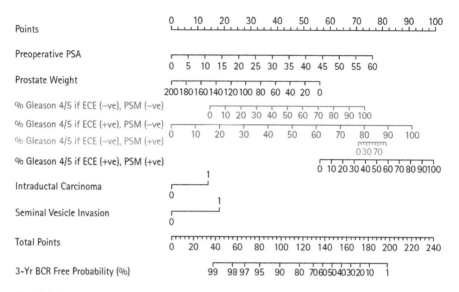

Fig. 8.4 Postoperative nomogram predicting 3-year BCR-free probability after RP [Reprinted with permission of John Wiley and Sons, Publishers, from O'Brien et al. (2010)]

final model, we see, for example, that preoperative serum PSA level (PSA), the presence of intraductal carcinoma (IDCP), and seminal vesicle invasion (SVI) are all positively associated with the risk of BCR, with hazard ratios of 1.05, 1.72, and 1.98, respectively. For example, invasion of the carcinoma into the seminal vesicles virtually doubles the hazard of BCR, controlling for other factors. On the other hand, greater prostate weight is associated with a lower risk of BCR (hazard ratio = 0.99). This final model has excellent prognostic accuracy (i.e., discriminatory power), with a c index value of 0.828.

Interpreting the effects of the variables % 4/5, PSM, and ECE is not quite as straightforward, because these variables interact with each other. How do we interpret, for example, the effect of % 4/5? Because of the interaction effects, the hazard ratio for % 4/5 is expressed as

$$(1.03)(0.98^{PSM})(1.012^{ECE}).$$

That is, this hazard ratio, which is the multiplicative effect of an increasing percent of Gleason grade 4/5 tumors on BCR, is multiplied by two other terms that are functions of positive surgical margins and extracapsular extension, respectively. In other words, the effect of % 4/5 depends on the values of both PSM and ECE simultaneously. This is taken account of in the predictive nomogram, which is shown in Fig. 8.4. Note that the nomogram predicts 3-year survival probability, that is, the probability of surviving BCR-free for 3 years after radical prostatectomy.

In the authors' figure legend, they explain how to use the nomogram (p. 394):

A patient's points for the variables preoperative PSA, prostate weight, IDCP and SVI are calculated by drawing a line up from the scale bar for each variable to the points bar at the top. To calculate the points for % Gleason 4/5, the correct color-coded [color not reproduced here] scale bar is selected by taking into account the patient's status for surgical margins and ECE. The points for all variables are then added to calculate total points. A line is drawn from the total points bar at the bottom of the nomogram to the probability bar below, giving the patient's predicted chance of remaining free of BCR at 3 years after RP.

Let's calculate a couple of survival probabilities using this nomogram. In particular, let's try to understand how the effect of % 4/5 depends on PSM and ECE. Suppose that a patient has preoperative PSA of 20, prostate weight of 120, no Intraductal Carcinoma (IDCP = 0), and Seminal Vesicle Invasion (SVI = 1). And then let's consider the effect of % 4/5 by assessing the change in the survival probability if the patient has 40 % Gleason 4/5 vs. 30 % Gleason 4/5. In other words, we examine the effect of an increase of 10 % in Gleason 4/5 on survival probability. But we do this under two different conditions: Case 1: a patient with ECE (−ve), PSM (−ve); Case 2: a patient with ECE (+ve), PSM (+ve). The points for a Case 1 patient with 30 % Gleason 4/5 are 25 (PSA), 22.5 (prostate weight), 0 (IDCP), 17.5 (SVI), and 32 (Gleason 4/5) for a total of 97. The points for a Case 1 patient with 40 % Gleason 4/5 are 25 (PSA), 22.5 (prostate weight), 0 (IDCP), 17.5 (SVI), and 37.5 (Gleason 4/5), for a total of 102.5. The corresponding survival probabilities are 0.91 for 30 % 4/5 and 0.89 for 40 % 4/5. The difference is approximately 0.02. Hence, a 10 % increase in Gleason 4/5 at this setting of ECE and PSM translates into a reduction of 0.02 in the survival probability.

For Case 2, the only mathematical changes are with respect to the % 4/5 values. The points are 67.5 for 30 % Gleason 4/5 and 72.5 for 40 % Gleason 4/5. The total points are then 132.5 and 137.5 for 30 % 4/5 and 40 % 4/5, respectively. The corresponding survival probabilities are 0.67 and 0.60, respectively. The reduction in survival probability due to a 10 % increase in % 4/5 in this case is 0.07. What we've shown, then, is that the reduction in survival probability due to increasing the percent of Gleason grade 4/5 cancer by 10 % is 0.02 at one setting of ECE and PSM values and 0.07 at a different setting of those values. This means that the "effect" of % 4/5 on BCR depends on ECE and PSM, which is exactly the meaning of an interaction effect. Hopefully this exercise has also illustrated how to effectively use this device for prognostic purposes.

Finally, the authors comment on a study limitation, as well as the particular usefulness of their nomogram for identifying at-risk patients (p. 394):

One of the main limitations of our study is the short follow-up times for BCR-free patients, which limits our nomogram to predicting BCR-free survival at 3 years post-RP. This has occurred because patients remaining BCR free at 2–3 years after RP are commonly referred back to their GPs for follow-up, but these PSA results are seldom forwarded to the treating urologists for our data collection purposes unless the patient develops BCR. We hope to rectify this problem in the future. However, research shows that 45–58% of BCRs occur within 2 years of surgery [25,26] and that patients developing BCR within 2 years are significantly more likely to progress to metastasis within 3–5 years of BCR [25]. Our nomogram will be useful for predicting these potentially ominous early failures, thus identifying patients who may benefit from adjuvant therapy.

Survival Following Radical Cystectomy

Yafi and colleagues (2010) studied factors related to various types of survival after patients had undergone radical cystectomy (RC). The sample consisted of 2,287 (21.2 % female) patients who underwent RC at eight different academic centers across Canada between 1998 and 2008. Three different study endpoints were examined: overall survival (OS), recurrence-free survival (RFS), and disease-specific survival (DSS). Overall survival time refers to the time interval from RC until death due to any cause. Recurrence-free survival is the time interval from RC until the first evidence of clinical recurrence of bladder cancer. Disease-specific survival pertains to the time interval from RC to death specifically from bladder cancer. In this last analysis, patients who died from causes other than bladder cancer were considered censored as of the time of death. Also considered censored at time of death in this analysis were patients succumbing to perioperative mortality, defined by the authors as death within 30 days of surgery or before discharge home (Yafi et al. 2010). Cox regression results for the outcomes OS and DSS are shown in Table 8.7.

Of the demographic and lifestyle factors at the top of the table, smoking is a significant predictor of survival after surgery, even controlling for critical clinical factors. The hazard ratio of 1.3 suggests that smoking raises the hazard of death by about 30 % overall. Smoking also raises the hazard of death due specifically to bladder cancer by the same amount. The authors highlight this effect as an important contribution of the study (p. 543):

> This is the first report on the impact of smoking on DSS following RC for bladder cancer, thus further emphasizing the deleterious associations of smoking not only with increasing bladder cancer incidence, but also with cancer-specific outcomes following curative surgical intervention.

Interestingly, adjuvant chemotherapy reduces the hazard of death overall by about 30 %, a very significant effect ($p < 0.001$). Although it is also estimated to reduce the hazard of death due to bladder cancer by about 25 %, this latter effect is not quite significant ($p = 0.056$).

PSA Doubling Time and Metastasis After Radical Prostatectomy

Antonarakis and fellow researchers (2011) examined metastasis-free survival after radical prostatectomy (RP). Their primary explanatory variable was the time it takes for PSA readings to double in men with PSA recurrence following RP. The authors cited prior research pointing to the importance of PSA doubling time as a risk factor for metastasis. The sample was described by the authors as follows (p. 33):

> Of all men undergoing radical prostatectomy at Johns Hopkins Hospital between July 1981 and July 2010, 1973 developed biochemical recurrence (defined as a postoperative PSA ≥ 0.2 ng/mL). After eliminating patients who received adjuvant/neoadjuvant or salvage therapies

Table 8.7 Univariate and multivariate cox regression analyses of clinical and pathological variables for predicting overall and disease-specific survival following radical cystectomy [Reprinted with Permission of John Wiley and Sons, Publishers, from Yafi et al. (2010)]

	Univariate analysis OS	Multivariate analysis OS			Univariate analysis DSS	Multivariate analysis DSS		
	p	HR	95 % CI	p	p	HR	95 % CI	p
Age	0.001	1.012	1.001–1.023	0.025	0.755	1.002	0.990–1.014	0.777
Gender	0.445	1.246	0.982–1.583	0.071	0.233	1.209	0.911–1.605	0.189
Smoking	0.004	1.307	1.049–1.628	0.017	0.031	1.304	1.005–1.691	0.046
Diversion								
Ileal conduit		Reference				Reference		
Other	0.009	0.723	0.536–0.795	0.034	0.216	0.723	0.514–1.018	0.063
PLND								
PLND		Reference				Reference		
None	0.1	1.406	0.937–2.108	0.100	0.007	1.709	1.084–2.693	0.021
Pathological stage								
≤P2		Reference				Reference		
>P2	<0.001	2.119	1.591–2.823	<0.001	<0.001	2.390	1.669–3.422	<0.001
Pathological nodal status								
PN−		Reference				Reference		
PN+	<0.001	2.335	1.860–2.930	<0.001	<0.001	2.765	2.124–3.600	<0.001
Grade	0.001	0.885	0.622–1.261	0.500	<0.001	0.892	0.585–1.361	0.596
Histology								
TCC		Reference				Reference		
Non-TCC	0.006	0.764	0.506–1.154	0.201	0.027	0.758	0.466–1.234	0.265
Margins	<0.001	2.033	1.538–2.689	<0.001	<0.001	2.312	1.685–3.172	<0.001
Adjuvant chemotherapy	0.004	0.705	0.541–0.919	0.0100	<0.001	0.747	0.554–1.007	0.056

DSS disease-specific survival, *HR* hazard ratio, *OS* overall survival, *PLND* pelviclymph node dissection, *TCC* transitional cell carcinoma

Stratification by PSA doubling time

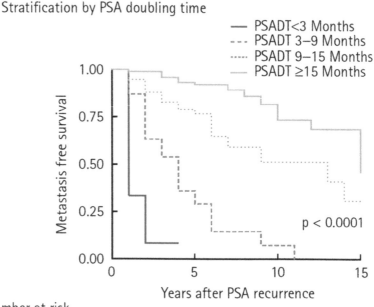

mber at risk

Fig. 8.5 Survival curves for metastasis-free survival stratified by PSA doubling time (PSADT) [Reprinted with permission of John Wiley and Sons, Publishers, from Antonarakis et al. (2011)]

before the detection of metastases ($n = 798$), and excluding patients with other missing information ($n = 533$), 642 men remained (Fig. 1). Only 450 men had sufficient data to allow calculation of PSADT, and these patients alone formed our cohort. Patients were followed through December 2010.

Metastatic disease was defined as "the presence of osseous metastases on bone scan, or visceral (liver, lung, brain) or extra-pelvic nodal metastases on CT scan" (Antonarakis et al. 2011, p. 34). The study endpoint was metastasis-free survival (MFS), defined as "the time interval from biochemical recurrence to initial metastasis" (Antonarakis et al. 2011, p. 34). At last follow-up, 29.4 % of patients had developed metastases (Antonarakis et al. 2011, p. 35). PSA doubling time was calculated as described by the authors (p. 34):

PSADT was calculated using the log of 2 divided by the slope of the linear regression line of the log of PSA value against time (in months). All PSA values ≥ 0.2 ng/mL obtained within 24 months after biochemical recurrence were used. A minimum of two PSA levels collected ≥ 3 months apart were required. Because no patient received salvage therapy upon biochemical recurrence, PSADT determinations were not influenced by treatment.

The authors employed Kaplan–Meier estimates of survival functions, stratified by selected prognostic factors, for a preliminary look at how prognostic factors affected MFS. Multivariable analyses were then done with the Cox model.

Figure 8.5 shows how MFS differs according to PSA doubling time using the Kaplan–Meier method. The p value for the log rank test is shown in the lower right corner of the figure.

Table 8.8 Cox proportional hazards models for MFS [Reprinted with permission of John Wiley and Sons, Publishers, from Antonarakis et al. (2011)]

	Univariate model		Multivariable model	
Variables	HR (95 % CI)	p	HR (95 % CI)	p
Age at surgery, years (continuous)	0.99 (0.96–1.02)	0.713	1.01 (0.98–1.04)	0.464
Race				
White	1 [reference]		1 [reference]	
Non-white	0.4 (0.2–0.8)	0.010	0.5 (0.2–1.1)	0.086
Preoperative PSA, ng/mL (continuous)	1.00 (0.99–1.01)	0.567	0.99 (0.98–1.01)	0.424
Pathological Gleason sum				
4–6	1 [reference]		1 [reference]	
7	4.3 (1.7–10.7)	0.002	2.4 (0.9–6.2)	0.067
8–10	10.9 (4.4–27.1)	<0.001	4.5 (1.7–11.9)	0.002
Pathological stage				
Organ-confined disease	1 [reference]		1 [reference]	
Extraprostatic extension	1.2 (0.6–2.3)	0.658	0.6 (0.3–1.3)	0.240
Seminal vesicle invasion	3.0 (1.5–6.0)	0.002	1.3 (0.6–2.8)	0.434
Lymph node involvement	3.1 (1.6–6.0)	0.001	1.1 (0.5–2.2)	0.811
Surgical margin status				
Negative	1 [reference]		1 [reference]	
Positive	0.8 (0.6–1.1)	0.198	0.9 (0.6–1.4)	0.829
Time to PSA recurrence				
≤3 years	1 [reference]		1 [reference]	
>3 years	0.4 (0.3–0.6)	<0.001	1.0 (0.6–1.5)	0.964
PSA doubling time				
≥15 months	1 [reference]		1 [reference]	
9.0–14.9 months	2.7 (1.6–4.8)	0.005	2.5 (1.4–4.5)	0.002
3.0–8.9 months	11.6 (7.0–19.3)	<0.001	8.0 (4.5–14.1)	<0.001
<3.0 months	47.4 (25.2–89.0)	<0.001	33.3 (16.4–67.4)	<0.001

HR hazard ratio

The differences in survival curves according to PSADT are striking. The highest curve is for PSADT≥15 months, and the lowest is for PSADT<3 months. The log rank test is very significant ($p < 0.0001$), suggesting that survival curves are significantly different for men characterized by different values of PSADT.

Table 8.8 presents the results of univariate and multivariable Cox regression models for the hazard of metastasis.

In the multivariable model, we see that PSA doubling time still has a very significant effect on the hazard of metastasis, even after controlling for several other clinical factors. For example, those with doubling time under 3 months have 33 times the hazard of metastasis, compared to those with doubling time of 15 months or more ($p < 0.001$). We also notice that nonwhites have significantly lower hazard of metastasis at any given time in the univariate model (HR = 0.4, $p = 0.01$). But this effect is no longer quite significant in the multivariable model ($p = 0.086$). Apparently, the effect of race is partly accounted for by the association of race with clinical factors added into the multivariable model.

Race Differences in the Risk of Prostate Cancer

Pettaway and colleagues (2011) followed a cohort of African American and Caucasian men to assess the progression of prostate disease severity after a diagnosis of benign prostatic hyperplasia (BPH). Their sample consisted of all men aged 50–79 years who had been diagnosed with BPH in 1995 at the Henry Ford Health System in Detroit. The men were followed over an 11-year period. A main endpoint of the study was the development of prostate cancer (PC). The researchers were particularly interested in assessing whether African Americans might be at higher risk for the disease than Caucasians. They also examined the role of therapy with α-blockers (to control short-term symptoms) and 5α-reductase inhibitors (to reduce prostate size) in altering disease risk (Pettaway et al. 2011). In the following passage, the authors detail their exclusionary criteria and measurement of inception of risk (p. 1303; AUR refers to acute urinary retention):

> Men with a diagnosis of AUR within 1 day of study entry were considered to be prevalent cases at baseline and were excluded from the analysis. Similarly, men undergoing prostate surgery within 1 week of entry into the study and men with prostate cancer diagnosed within 6 months of enrolment were considered prevalent cases and excluded from their respective analyses...Time at risk of each outcome began at the time that cases identified ceased to be categorized as prevalent cases; that is, 1 day after study entry for AUR, 1 week after study entry for prostate surgery, and 6 months after study entry for prostate cancer.

Preliminary findings regarding a potential interaction between baseline PSA and race in their effects on the rate of PC are shown in Fig. 8.6.

The authors say (p. 1304) "There also appeared to be a potential interaction between race, PSA level and risk of prostate cancer..." In the figure, we see that for

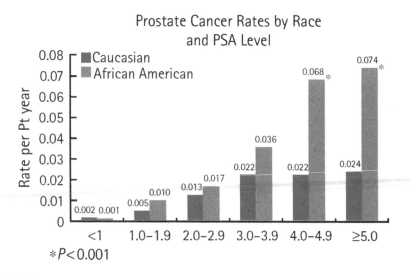

Fig. 8.6 Prostate cancer rates by race and baseline PSA [Reprinted with permission of John Wiley and Sons, Publishers, from Pettaway et al. (2011)]

Table 8.9 Cox regression model results for the risk of prostate cancer by race and other factors [Reprinted with permission of John Wiley and Sons, Publishers, from Pettaway et al. (2011)]

	Hazard ratio (95 % confidence interval)	p-Value
African American race	2.21 (1.47–3.33)	<0.001
Index age	1.02 (1.00–1.05)	0.033
Prostate-specific antigen	1.02 (1.01–1.02)	<0.001
Income		
Low income	1.	
Medium income	1.06 (0.49–2.28)	0.885
High income	1.68 (0.77–3.67)	0.191
Therapy		
α-blocker	1.07 (0.77–1.50)	0.674
5α-reductase	0.76 (0.28–2.09)	0.599

PSA under 1.0, there is no race difference in the rate of PC. But as PSA levels increase to 1.0–1.9, 2.0–2.9, etc., the rate of PC for African Americans appears to be greater than for Caucasians at each PSA level. At the two highest levels of PSA, the race difference is significant. For example, among men with PSA of 4.0–4.9, 6.8 % of African Americans vs. 2.2 % of Caucasians had developed PC. Among men with PSA of 5.0 or higher, 7.4 % of African Americans vs. 2.4 % of Caucasians had developed PC. From the article, it is unclear whether this interaction effect is significant; the authors mention no test for it. That the rates are significantly different by race in some categories of PSA but not others does not necessarily indicate a significant interaction. This is most likely why the authors' phrasing merely refers to the "appearance" of an interaction effect. We return to this issue shortly.

Cox regression results for the risk of PC are presented in Table 8.9. Here we see that the race difference in the hazard of PC is significant even after controlling for PSA, age, income, and therapeutic regimen. African Americans have a risk of developing PC that is over twice that of Caucasians (hazard ratio=2.21, $p<0.001$). We see, also, that older men are at higher risk for PC, as are those with higher PSA levels. Neither income nor therapeutic regimen has a significant effect on the development of PC. This analysis could easily have incorporated an interaction effect between race and PSA via the inclusion in the model of a crossproduct term taking the form "African American race × Prostate-specific antigen." Such a term would have allowed the testing of whether such an interaction effect was significant. However, the authors do not mention such a test, so it is unclear how much credence should be given to the suggested interaction shown in Fig. 8.6. Perhaps the research team will explore this issue further in subsequent studies.

In the next chapter, we will add a number of new techniques to the reader's statistical arsenal. Although the regression models covered so far are adequate for most medical research, cutting-edge developments in statistics have led to a host of specialized statistical tools coming into more frequent use. These techniques include Poisson and negative-binomial regression, propensity-score analysis, multiple imputation, growth-curve modeling, and fixed-effects regression modeling. The readers' statistical education would not be complete without them.

Chapter 9
Other Advanced Techniques

In this chapter we will learn about several additional advanced multivariate statistical techniques that are finding increasing application in medical research. *Multiple imputation* is a technique that allows us to "fill in" missing data. Often data on the study endpoint or the explanatory variables are missing for subjects in a study. If these subjects are therefore excluded from analysis, not only do we waste the data that they have provided, but their exclusion also introduces selection bias into the analyses. Multiple imputation allows us to fill in, or impute, the missing data with an estimate of what the data would have been had they been present. Once the data have been imputed, they can be used in any of the types of analyses that are discussed in this primer. *Poisson regression* and its close relative *negative binomial regression* are the appropriate models to employ when the study endpoint is a count of the number of events that have occurred to the subject in a given time period. Because counts must be represented by integer values and cannot be negative, we cannot use linear regression for this analysis, for reasons explained below. *Propensity-score analysis* is a statistical tool that allows us to mimic random assignment to "treatment categories," even though our data are from an observational study. Although we can control statistically for potentially confounding variables in an observational study, a problem arises if these covariates are imbalanced across groups. That is, the different treatment groups of interest have very different distributions on the covariates. Propensity-score analysis is designed to balance measured covariates across treatment groups in order to more effectively simulate random assignment to treatment. *Growth-curve modeling* is useful whenever people are studied over time and interest centers on the pattern of change in a quantitative study endpoint over that time period. Because people contribute multiple time points' worth of measurements to the analysis, linear regression is inadequate to model the complex error term required in these studies. Growth-curve models elegantly incorporate the additional complexity into their structure. Finally, we will consider the dilemma we began with in Chap. 1 involving latent selection factors. What happens if there are one or more unmeasured covariates that might be driving

A. DeMaris and S.H. Selman, *Converting Data into Evidence: A Statistics Primer for the Medical Practitioner*, DOI 10.1007/978-1-4614-7792-1_9,
© Springer Science+Business Media New York 2013

our results? *Fixed-effects regression modeling* is one technique that, under the right conditions, eliminates the threat from confounds that have not been measured. Several examples from the medical literature will help to illustrate the use of these important techniques.

Multiple Imputation

Missing data in medical studies is a perennial problem. People in clinical trials who are followed up over multiple time points may drop out of the study at some point. All of their response values from that point on are necessarily missing. In observational studies based on interviewing respondents, very often respondents do not provide answers to some of the items. They may not know the answer, deem it inapplicable to them, or simply refuse to respond. The end result of all these difficulties is that the data are missing on either the study endpoint or the independent variables for some portion of one's sample. Several simple "fixes" for the problem have been used in the past. One solution is to employ *listwise deletion*. This means that one eliminates from the sample all cases that are missing on any of the variables in the study. Although this approach has advantages in some situations (Allison 2002), it may result in a drastic reduction in one's sample size and a concomitant loss of statistical power (Johnson and Young 2011). Another simple solution is to replace the missing value with a number that constitutes one's best "guess" for the missing value. This might just be the mean value of the variable for all cases with valid values on the item, an approach referred to as *marginal mean imputation* (Allison 2002). A better solution in the same vein would be to regress the problematic variable on other independent variables at hand. Then one can use the resulting prediction equation to generate a predicted value for the case that is missing on that variable. This is known as *conditional mean imputation* (Allison 2002). Or, in a longitudinal study, missing values on the study endpoint may be replaced by the last observed value of the study endpoint. This approach is known as the *last observation carried forward* strategy (Green et al. 2009; Nickel et al. 2011). However, all of the aforementioned simple fixes are flawed. As mentioned, listwise deletion wastes data. Strategies that replace a missing value with a single number fail to take prediction error into account in the imputation (Allison 2002). Moreover, those that replace several missing values with the same number, as in marginal mean imputation, artificially reduce the variance in the affected variables (Allison 2002). What is the preferred strategy?

Currently, two procedures for dealing with missing data are considered optimum. One of these is *full-information maximum likelihood estimation* or FIML. This is a very complex procedure that sees limited use and will not be discussed at length here. Briefly, define the "incomplete data" as the complete dataset that includes all cases even though some of their data values are missing. In a nutshell, FIML derives the likelihood function for the parameters of one's model based on the incomplete data. The model parameters are then estimated by maximizing this particular likelihood function (see Little and Rubin 1987, or Allison 2002, for further details). The other approach sees widespread use in medical research, and as mentioned above, is called multiple imputation or MI. Two assumptions are typically made in using MI. The first is that one's cases, consisting of the measurement of a study endpoint and explanatory variables for each of one's analytic units, are observations drawn from a *multivariate normal distribution* (Little and Rubin 1987; Schafer 2000). This is a multidimensional version of the normal distribution that we discussed in Chap. 2. If a set of variables is characterized by a multivariate normal distribution, then each individual variable in the set has a normal distribution. Moreover, each variable can be written as a linear regression function of the other variables. That is, its mean follows a linear regression model with all of the other variables as its predictors. The second assumption is that the data are *missing at random*. This means that the probability a case has a missing value on a variable is independent of what the value of that variable would have been had it been observed (Allison 2002; Little and Rubin 1987). In other words, there is no tendency for those who, say, would have had lower values on the variable in question to be more likely to be missing on it.

Suppose that these assumptions are satisfied. Then when a variable in the dataset is missing for one or more cases, these values can be predicted from the corresponding linear regression function of the other variables. So suppose one has a study endpoint, Y, and the explanatory variables X_1, X_2, and X_3, for a sample of n cases. And suppose that Y and X_2 are missing for some of the cases. One can regress Y on X_1, X_2, and X_3 for all cases with valid values on these variables. Based on this regression equation, one can obtain predicted values of Y for the missing observations. The same can be done with X_2. We regress X_2 on Y, X_1, and X_3 for all those with valid observations and then use the regression equation to generate predicted values of X_2 for the missing observations. However, we don't stop there. To each predicted value is added a random error term to account for the uncertainty involved in the prediction. In this manner, we generate predicted values for all the missing data, and we have a complete dataset for analysis. And then the procedure is repeated using a different set of random errors to generate a different complete dataset for analysis. This is done again and again. The result is a collection of complete datasets, with each one distinguished by having somewhat different imputed values for the missing data. Researchers will typically generate anywhere from 5 to 50 complete datasets via the MI technique. With each dataset, one runs one's statistical analysis. So if the analysis is a regression of Y on X_1, X_2, and X_3 and we have 50 imputed datasets, we run the regression 50 times, each time using a different imputed dataset. When we're done, we combine all of the 50 sets of regression coefficients and all of the 50 sets of standard errors for those coefficients into one final set of coefficients and standard errors. Combining is done using a weighted averaging procedure, as discussed in Allison (2002) and Little and Rubin (1987). Then a test for the significance of each of these final coefficients is a t test consisting of each coefficient divided by its standard error (Allison 2002; Little and Rubin 1987). Although it may seem as though we are just making up data here, the procedure is fully justified by statistical theory (Allison 2002; Little and Rubin 1987; Schafer 2000). Moreover, it produces unbiased estimates of the parameters of interest.

Poisson and Negative-Binomial Regression

An *event count* is the *number of occurrences of an event within a fixed domain of observation* (King 1988). An *event* is a discrete occurrence, such as a heart attack, stroke, seizure, or other medical episode. The domain of observation is the time period during which the subject is observed. For example, Rosenfeld and colleagues (2012) conducted a multicenter clinical trial to examine whether the inhalation of hypertonic saline would diminish the number of pulmonary exacerbations in a sample of children suffering from cystic fibrosis. The event in question here was a pulmonary exacerbation, and the domain of observation was the time from randomization to treatment/placebo until the last in-clinic visit or follow-up telephone call. Children were followed for up to 48 weeks after randomization to treatment groups. The number of pulmonary exacerbations was the primary study endpoint in this trial. It is necessarily integer-valued, ranging from 0 to whatever the greatest number of exacerbations was observed in this sample. The domain of observation was the time period during which a given child was followed up, which varied for different children. Two model covariates were age category and study site (Rosenfeld et al. 2012). One way to approach the analysis of these data would be to use linear regression to regress the number of exacerbations on model covariates. However, that is not the optimum strategy when the study endpoint is a count. One reason is that a count cannot take on negative values. But the right-hand side of the linear regression equation is not constrained by that condition. It is free to take on any value. Hence, it is easy to get negative predicted counts using this modeling approach. Another problem is that the linear regression model assumes that the study endpoint is normally distributed at each combination of predictor values. Yet count data do not typically have a normal distribution; rather their distribution is usually right-skewed. The distribution that is most appropriate for a count variable, at least as a starting point, is the Poisson distribution. This distribution for any variable, X, has one parameter, μ, and is expressed as:

$$P(x) = \frac{\exp(-\mu)\mu^x}{x!},$$

where $P(x)$ is the probability associated with x, a particular value of the variable, and $x!$, pronounced "x factorial" is $x\,(x-1)\,(x-2)\,(x-3)...(2)\,(1)$. (For example, $5! = (5)\,(4)\,(3)\,(2)\,(1) = 120$.) By specifying the value of the parameter μ, we can find the probability associated with any value of x. So if μ is 1.25, for example, then the probability that x equals 3 is:

$$P(3) = \frac{\exp(-1.25)1.25^3}{3!} = 0.093.$$

On the other hand, the probability that x equals 5 is:

$$P(5) = \frac{\exp(-1.25)1.25^5}{5!} = 0.007.$$

The parameter μ is both the mean and the variance of X in this distribution (DeMaris 2004).

The Poisson regression model assumes that Y has a Poisson distribution, in which the mean, μ, is influenced by one's explanatory variables. This Poisson distribution is used as the basis for maximum likelihood estimation of the regression coefficients (DeMaris 2004). Moreover, the regression model employs $\log(\mu)$ as the response. That is, the model is for the log of the mean of Y. The reason for this is theoretical (see, e.g., Cameron and Trivedi 1998; DeMaris 2004). But it also has the advantage of ensuring that predicted values of μ are nonnegative. The Poisson regression model is:

$$\log(\mu) = \alpha + \beta_1 X_1 + \beta_2 X_2 + \ldots + \beta_K X_K. \tag{9.1}$$

It resembles a linear regression model except that the response is the log of the mean of Y. The Poisson regression model has one drawback, however. The conditional mean and variance have to be the same value, as they are essentially the same parameter. In practice, the variance of Y often exceeds its mean, thereby violating this assumption of the Poisson specification. If this is the case, standard errors of coefficients will not be correct; they will typically be underestimated. This means that we will be falsely inclined to declare predictor effects "significant" in the model, when their true effects are nil. A remedy for this problem is to use the *negative binomial distribution* to represent the distribution of Y. The difference between it and the Poisson distribution is that the former incorporates an extra parameter. This is called the *overdispersion* parameter. It allows the variance to exceed the mean and results in better estimates and more accurate standard errors. The negative binomial regression model looks exactly like the Poisson regression model, above. The only difference is the presence of the overdispersion parameter, which is contained in the likelihood function for maximum likelihood estimation. We do not see it in the regression equation itself. Moreover, we can test whether the overdispersion parameter itself is significant. If it is not, then the Poisson model is to be preferred.

Coefficients for Poisson or negative binomial regression are both interpreted the same way. They can be seen as effects on the log of the mean of Y. However, a more convenient way of talking about them is afforded by exponentiating them. To understand the rationale for this, let us exponentiate both sides of (9.1):

$$\text{Exp}[\log(\mu)] = \exp[\alpha + \beta_1 X_1 + \beta_2 X_2 + \ldots + \beta_K X_K]$$

or:

$$\mu = \exp(\alpha)\exp(\beta_1 X_1)\exp(\beta_2 X_2)\ldots\exp(\beta_K X_K)$$

or:

$$\mu = \exp(\alpha)\exp(\beta_1)^{X_1}\exp(\beta_2)^{X_2}\ldots\exp(\beta_K)^{X_K}. \tag{9.2}$$

Equation (9.2) makes it clear that $\exp(\beta_1)$, for example, is the *multiplicative impact* on the mean of Y for each unit increase in X_1, controlling for the other Xs in the model. The other coefficients are similarly interpreted. Sometimes the Poisson or negative binomial model is couched as a model for the *rate of event occurrence*. We define the average rate of occurrence as the average number of events divided by the domain of observation. Let D represent the domain of observation. A Poisson model for the rate of event occurrences is then:

$$\frac{\mu}{D} = \exp(\alpha)\exp(\beta_1)^{X_1}\exp(\beta_2)^{X_2}\ldots\exp(\beta_K)^{X_K}$$

or:

$$\mu = D\exp(\alpha)\exp(\beta_1)^{X_1}\exp(\beta_2)^{X_2}\ldots\exp(\beta_K)^{X_K}$$

and due to the identity $D = \text{Exp}[\log(D)]$, we have

$$\mu = \exp(\log(D))\exp(\alpha)\exp(\beta_1)^{X_1}\exp(\beta_2)^{X_2}\ldots\exp(\beta_K)^{X_K}$$

or with the log of μ as the response:

$$\log(\mu) = \alpha + \log(D) + \beta_1 X_1 + \beta_2 X_2 + \ldots + \beta_K X_K. \tag{9.3}$$

Equation (9.3) shows that the rate of event occurrence is easily modeled by including the log of the domain size as an extra predictor. However, its coefficient is constrained to equal 1. This type of variable in either the Poisson or negative binomial regression model is referred to as an *offset* (DeMaris 2004). A substantive example will aid in our understanding of this technique.

An Illustrative Example: Pregnancy Stress in the NAPPS Study

Illustrative data for this chapter were drawn from the New Arrivals: Passage to Parenthood Study (NAPPS; DeMaris et al. 2010, 2011; Mahoney et al. 2009). The initial sample consisted of 178 married couples experiencing the third trimester of pregnancy of both spouse's first biological child. They were drawn from a mid-sized, Midwestern city and surrounding suburban and rural communities. Couples were recruited via childbirth classes; announcements posted in medical offices, retail locations, or newspapers; word of mouth referrals; or direct mail. Inclusionary criteria were that spouses: (a) were married, (b) pregnant with each individual's first biological child, and (c) spoke English. Data were collected in couples' homes. Each spouse independently completed surveys that assessed the constructs used in the study. A research assistant was present throughout, both to answer any questions

Table 9.1 Linear, poisson, and negative-binomial regression coefficients for the regression of number of pregnancy stressors on explanatory variables

Explanatory variable	Linear regression	Poisson regression	Negative-binomial regression
Intercept	4.371**	1.508***	1.506***
Unintended pregnancy	0.415	0.069	0.069
Age	0.103	0.017	0.017
Household income (in thousands)	−0.012	−0.002	−0.002
Number of years married	−0.220	−0.037*	−0.037*
Work hours	−0.004	−0.001	−0.001
Relative advantage	0.267***	0.043***	0.042***
Dispersion parameter			0.025
R^2	0.121	0.135	0.135

* $p<.05$; ** $p<.01$; *** $p<.001$

and to ensure that spouses completed the surveys independently. Couples were reassessed in the same manner three more times over the course of the next year: at 4, 7, and 13 months after the first visit. These constitute waves 2–4 of the study and encompass approximately the first full year of the life of the newborn. Couples were paid $75.00, $100.00, $100.00, and $125.00 for their participation in waves 1–4, respectively. Data collection began in October, 2005 and ended in August, 2008.

The study endpoint for Poisson/negative binomial regression was the *number of pregnancy stressors* experienced. This was asked of mothers in wave 1 of the survey. They were asked to check any of "the following difficulties that you may have experienced throughout your pregnancy." This was followed by a number of problems that were both physical ("spotting," "back pain," "recurrent urinary tract infections") and emotional ("loss of control over emotions," "criticism/lack of support from family or friends about pregnancy"). The range of the stressor index was from 1 to 16 reported difficulties, with a mean of 5.9 and a standard deviation of 2.8. The primary explanatory variable in the analyses in this chapter was *unintended pregnancy*, coded 1 if the pregnancy was unintended, and 0 if it was intended, based on both husband's and wife's responses. An unintended pregnancy was defined as a pregnancy that was either unwanted—the couple did not want to have a child—or mistimed, in particular, occurring earlier than intended (Zolna and Lindberg 2012). Forty-six percent of the pregnancies were not intended at the time they occurred. Other predictors of interest, all measured in wave 1, were mother's *age*, *household income* in thousands of dollars, *number of years the couple was married*, *number of hours per week the mother worked outside the home*, and mother's *relative advantage*. This last was the mother's perception regarding the balance of contributions to the marital relationship on the part of each spouse. The higher the score, the greater the mother's perception that her husband was contributing more than she was (DeMaris et al. 2010). Table 9.1 presents the results of three different regression models for the number of pregnancy stressors: linear regression estimated with ordinary least squares, Poisson regression, and negative binomial regression.

The linear regression identifies only one significant predictor: the relative advantage scale. Both the Poisson and negative binomial regressions identify two significant predictors: the relative advantage scale and the number of years married. The Poisson and negative binomial analyses are more to be trusted in this case, as they are more appropriate for a count variable. There is no need for an offset in this example, as the domain for all mothers was the same: the first 6 months of the pregnancy. Which is better: Poisson or negative binomial? The dispersion parameter's value is 0.025 but it is not significant. This suggests that the assumption of the Poisson model that the mean and variance of the study endpoint are the same is not violated. Hence, the Poisson model would seem to be most appropriate, although the results are quite comparable for both. The Poisson results are best interpreted by exponentiating the significant coefficients. Controlling for other factors, each additional year married reduces the average number of pregnancy stressors by a factor of $\exp(-0.037) = 0.964$ or by about 3.6 %. On the other hand, each unit increase in relative advantage increases the average number of pregnancy stressors by a factor of $\exp(0.043) = 1.044$, or by about 4.4 %. DeMaris and colleagues (2010) have found that women, in particular, tend to be distressed by being overbenefited. Although the effect of an unintended pregnancy on the pregnancy stressor index is positive, it is nowhere near significant ($p > 0.3$, not shown). The R^2 for the Poisson model indicates that about 13.5 % of the variance in number of pregnancy stressors is accounted for by the model.

Propensity Score Analysis

In nonexperimental studies, ANCOVA is typically used to reduce bias in the estimate of a "treatment" effect due to preexisting differences between treatment groups (Schafer and Kang 2008). However, among other things, the efficacy of ANCOVA in producing an unbiased estimate of a treatment effect rests on there being sufficient overlap in covariate distributions between treatment groups. Otherwise, the treatment-effect estimate is based on extrapolation to a hypothetical set of covariate values that may not represent any real cases (Schafer and Kang 2008). The result is a badly biased estimate of the treatment effect. The problem is illustrated in Fig. 9.1:

Shown is a scatterplot of Y with X for $n = 16$ cases. The treatment group is represented by the symbol "1" and the nontreatment, or control, group by the symbol "0." It is clear that the mean of Y for the treatment group, which is 14.8, is greater than the mean of Y for the control group, which is 6.45. The unadjusted mean difference on Y between groups is therefore $14.8 - 6.45 = 8.35$. We see, also, that the two groups have very different distributions on the covariate, X. The mean of X for the control group is 2.8, and for the treatment group it's 7.6. The ANCOVA model for Y is:

$$\hat{y} = 3.70 + 3.69\,\text{Treatment} + 0.98X.$$

Fig. 9.1 Plot of Y with X showing nonoverlap of X values for treatment ("trt"=1) and nontreatment ("trt"=0) groups

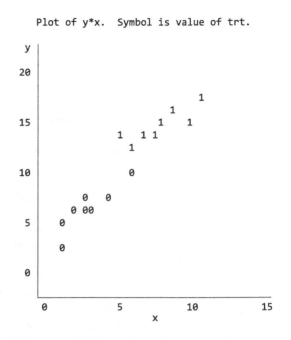

Plot of y*x. Symbol is value of trt.

It is clear from Fig. 9.1 and this equation that X has a strong positive linear effect on Y with a regression coefficient of 0.98 ($p<0.0001$). In the ANCOVA, the treatment effect is 3.69. This suggests that, controlling for differences on X, the mean difference is reduced from 8.35 to just 3.69. But how reliable is this? There is almost no overlap in the distribution on X for the two groups. That is, almost all X values in the control group are <5, and all X values in the treatment group are >5. What does it mean to say, "controlling for X" in this instance, when almost no case in the control group has the same X value as a case in the treatment group? As mentioned in Chap. 6, in ANCOVA it is customary to show adjusted means on Y for the treatment groups, adjusted for differences in the covariate distributions. This is usually done by holding X constant at its overall mean, which, in this example, is 5.2, and then using the ANCOVA equation to obtain predicted means. The adjusted means for treatment and control groups are:

$$\text{Treatment}: \bar{y}_{adj} = 3.70 + 3.69 + 0.98(5.2) = 12.49,$$

$$\text{Control}: \bar{y}_{adj} = 3.70 + 0.98(5.2) = 8.80.$$

The difference in adjusted means is the adjusted difference of 3.69. This, supposedly, is the treatment effect after "adjusting for X." But notice that it is based on a value of X (i.e., $X=5.2$) for which there are virtually *no cases*. We are therefore extrapolating outside the range of most of the observed responses. The resulting estimate is not very robust. The problem is compounded by having several imbalanced covariates in one's model, as is typically the case. Propensity scores are designed to redress the imbalance in covariate distributions across groups and thereby produce a more robust estimate of the treatment effect.

The following definition and justification of propensity scores draw heavily from the excellent article by Schafer and Kang (2008). A propensity score is the *conditional probability of receiving the treatment given the covariates*. Theoretically, treated and untreated cases with identical propensity scores would have identical distributions on the explanatory variables that were used to estimate the propensities. This suggests that cases with the same propensity score can be treated as though they were randomly assigned to treatment and control groups. Their mean difference on the study endpoint is therefore an estimate of the average causal effect of treatment for those cases. There is, of course, one caveat here. Propensity scores adjust for differences in *measured* covariates only. The assumption is that there is no unmeasured confound, or latent selection factor, that still distinguishes groups with the same propensity score (Guo and Fraser 2010; Schafer and Kang 2008). If this assumption is satisfied, then propensity-score analysis may be justified. Propensity scores can be estimated with a logistic regression of treatment status (coded 1 for treatment and 0 for control) on the covariates in one's study. The estimated propensities are the estimated probabilities of being in the treatment group, based on the logistic regression equation. One means of testing whether propensity-score analysis is to be preferred over ANCOVA is as follows. Estimate a logistic regression equation for treatment status using the covariates. Obtain the predicted logits, i.e., $\log[p/(1-p)]$, for each subject. Calculate the mean predicted logit in the treatment vs. the control group. Calculate the pooled (i.e., weighted average) standard deviation of the logits for the treatment vs. the control group. If the difference between the mean logits exceeds one-half of the pooled standard deviation of the logits, then causal inferences using ANCOVA are not trustworthy and propensity scores should be used (Rubin 2001; Schafer and Kang 2008).

An Example: Unintended Pregnancy and Mothers' Depression

We draw once again from the NAPPS study to illustrate propensity-score analysis. The study endpoint this time is *mothers' depression*. This measure employs ten items from the Center for Epidemiological Studies Depression Scale or CES-D (Mirowsky and Ross 1984). In all four waves of the study, mothers were asked to indicate how often they experienced certain feelings in the past week. Example items are "I was bothered by things that usually don't bother me," and "I felt that everything I did was an effort." Response choices ranged from "Rarely or none of the time (<1 day)" to "All of the time (5–7 days)," and were coded 0–3, respectively. The scale score ranged from 0 to 30 and had an alpha reliability ranging from 0.70 to 0.78 across the four waves of the study. (*Alpha reliability*, or Chronbach's alpha, ranges from 0 to 1 and indicates the proportion of a measure's variability that reflects a stable underlying trait; values above 0.70 are considered ideal.) For this example,

Table 9.2 Means on model covariates for those with intended vs. unintended pregnancies

Model covariate	Intended pregnancy	Unintended pregnancy	p-Value for mean difference
Age	28.083	26.122	0.0009
Household Income (in thousands)	66.880	55.793	0.0037
Number of years married	3.181	1.974	<0.0001
Education	6.000	5.817	0.1559
Number of pregnancy stressors	5.604	6.281	0.1105
Child is male	0.460	0.462	0.9811

Table 9.3 ANOVA and ANCOVA estimates and p-values for mothers' depression at wave 1

Explanatory variables	ANOVA	p-Value	ANCOVA	p-Value
Intercept	7.781	<0.0001	6.544	0.0238
Unintended pregnancy	2.255	0.0003	1.929	0.0020
Age			−0.026	0.7847
Household income (in thousands)			0.004	0.7510
Number of years married			0.059	0.7172
Education			−0.193	0.6076
Number of pregnancy stressors			0.536	<0.0001
Child is male			−0.635	0.2779
R^2	0.072		0.206	

we use only the wave 1 depression score. Theoretically, we expect that mothers whose pregnancy was unintended will experience more depression than others. As their pregnancy was not planned for that particular time, they should experience more distress about its consequences for their bodies or their personal adjustment. Model covariates are: mother's age and education, household income, number of years married, number of pregnancy stressors, and whether the fetus is male. Table 9.2 shows the distributions on these covariates for those with an intended, vs. an unintended, pregnancy.

We see that pregnancy-status groups have significantly different distributions— i.e., means—on three covariates: age, household income, and number of years married. The intended pregnancy mothers are older, have a higher household income, and have been married longer than the unintended pregnancy group. This may be a situation warranting propensity-score analysis. Nevertheless, we begin by using the traditional ANOVA/ANCOVA approach, regressing mother's depression first on a dummy variable for the pregnancy being unintended, then adding the other covariates. Table 9.3 presents these results.

We see in the ANOVA that those with an unintended pregnancy are, on average, about two-and-a-quarter units higher on depression than those whose pregnancies were intended ($p = 0.0003$). As a standard deviation of mother's depression is 4.2 (not shown), this is about a half of a standard deviation difference in depression, not a trivial amount. The other model covariates are included in the ANCOVA model shown in the last two columns of the table. Of the added covariates, the number of

Table 9.4 Logistic
regression estimates for
prediction of unintended
pregnancy for the purpose
of creating propensity scores

Explanatory variable	b	p-Value
Intercept	2.015	0.1830
Age	−0.044	0.4112
Household income (in thousands)	−0.009	0.1742
Number of years married	−0.280	0.0043
Education	0.051	0.8058
Model χ^2	22.037	0.0002
Hosmer–Lemeshow χ^2	14.062	0.0802
AUC	0.704	
Pseudo- R_1^2	0.116	
Pseudo- R_2^2	0.160	

pregnancy stressors, not surprisingly, has a very significant positive effect on depression. Each additional stressor adds about a half of a unit to average depression. Controlling for pregnancy stress and the other covariates, the effect of an unintended pregnancy is reduced somewhat, but is still quite significant ($p=0.002$). Is this a reliable finding? We turn to propensity-score analysis to check.

To estimate propensity scores, we use only the covariates that could presumably be causally antecedent to the pregnancy: mother's age and education, household income, and number of years married. Table 9.4 shows the results of the logistic regression model used to estimate propensity scores.

Apparently, the only significant predictor of unintended pregnancy status is the number of years married, which has a negative effect. Thus, the longer the couple has been married, the less likely the pregnancy was unintended. The Hosmer–Lemeshow chi-squared is not significant, suggesting that the model has an adequate fit. The AUC, at 0.704, also suggests a model with adequate predictive efficacy. According to Pseudo- R_1^2, the model accounts for about 11.6 % of the variance in pregnancy status, presuming that it is an either-or proposition. On the other hand, should one consider the intendedness of a pregnancy to be a continuous quantitative underlying variable, Pseudo- R_2^2 suggests that about 16 % of its variance is accounted for by the model. We then assessed whether propensity-score analysis was warranted. The mean logit for the unintended pregnancy group was −0.4473, and for the intended pregnancy group was 0.0894. The difference was 0.0894−(−0.4473)=0.5367. The pooled standard deviation of the logits was 0.7483, half of which was 0.374. As this is less than the mean difference of the logits, it appears that propensity-score analysis is warranted.

Using Propensity Scores

There are several ways to employ propensity scores once they are estimated (see, e.g., Guo and Fraser 2010; Schafer and Kang 2008). However, Schafer and Kang's extensive simulation study suggests that one particularly reliable technique is

Table 9.5 Crosstabulation of tercile of propensity scores with unintended pregnancy status

Tercile of propensity score	Intended pregnancy	Unintended pregnancy	Total
1	38	15	53
2	33	21	54
3	25	46	71
Total	96	82	178

subclassification, or *stratification*, by propensity scores. This approach has the advantage that it is easily accomplished using conventional software. The principle is simple. We begin by dividing the sample up into groups that have approximately comparable propensity scores. Normally, this would be done by categorizing the sample by quintiles (i.e., fifths) of the distribution of propensity scores. However, in the current example, this produced propensity-score groups with too few cases in either the intended or unintended pregnancy categories. For example, the second quintile only had nine in the unintended group, and the fifth quintile only had six in the intended group. Therefore, we used terciles (i.e., thirds) instead of quintiles to divide up the sample. Table 9.5 shows the cross-classification of tercile of the propensity-score distribution with pregnancy status for the 178 mothers in the sample:

As is evident, some of the cells are still a little thin. There are only 15 mothers in tercile 1 and 21 in tercile 2 with an unintended pregnancy. But these numbers are adequate for our purposes here.

It is always important to examine whether balance has been achieved in model covariate distributions for those in the same propensity-score category. Table 9.6 presents tests of mean differences, once again, for the model covariates, separately by tercile of propensity score.

There are no significant differences on the distributions of the model covariates for terciles 1 and 2. However, in tercile 3, significant differences obtained for number of years married and mother's education, with the intended group being higher on both factors. Nevertheless, overall, greater balance across model covariates has been achieved by grouping on propensity scores.

Once the terciles (or quintiles or even finer divisions) have been established, the procedure is simple. Within each propensity-score category, we examine the mean difference in the study endpoint by treatment group. Or, we can do an ANCOVA within each propensity-score category, controlling for important model covariates (Schafer and Kang 2008). The latter is the strategy used here. In that the number of pregnancy stressors was the most important covariate for mother's depression; we regressed depression on pregnancy status and number of pregnancy stressors separately for each tercile of propensity scores. The results are shown in Table 9.7, where only the effect of an unintended pregnancy is displayed.

It is evident that the coefficient for unintended pregnancy is positive in each tercile, although it is only significant in tercile 2 and marginally so in tercile 3. At this point, to combine these separate estimates into an overall effect, we simply calculate a weighted average of them. The proportions of the sample falling into each

Table 9.6 Mean differences on model covariates for those with intended vs. unintended pregnancies by tercile of propensity scores

Model covariate	Intended pregnancy	Unintended pregnancy	p-Value for mean difference
1 Tercile			
Age	31.026	29.800	0.2351
Household income (in thousands)	86.414	85.500	0.9254
Number of years married	4.790	4.817	0.9672
Education	6.105	6.333	0.3412
Number of pregnancy stressors	5.921	5.733	0.8238
Child is male	0.526	0.400	0.4073
2 Tercile			
Age	27.333	28.048	0.3832
Household income (in thousands)	64.886	69.286	0.4789
Number of years married	2.631	2.298	0.2688
Education	5.939	6.191	0.2920
Number of pregnancy stressors	5.121	5.905	0.2919
Child is male	0.485	0.381	0.4538
3 Tercile			
Age	24.600	24.043	0.3977
Household income (in thousands)	47.500	39.946	0.1139
Number of years married	1.460	0.899	0.0007
Education	5.920	5.478	0.0353
Number of pregnancy stressors	5.760	6.630	0.2433
Child is male	0.520	0.609	0.4699

Table 9.7 Coefficients for unintended pregnancy effect from ANCOVAs by tercile of propensity scores

Tercile	Coefficient	Standard error	T value	p Value
1	0.624	1.212	0.510	0.6091
2	2.950	1.074	2.750	0.0083
3	1.729	0.904	1.910	0.0599

tercile, which are 0.30, 0.30, and 0.40, respectively, are used as the weights. A weighted average of the coefficients is:

$$b = 0.30(0.624) + 0.30(2.950) + 0.40(1.729) = 1.76.$$

To combine the standard errors, we take a weighted average of the coefficient variances (which are just the squares of the standard errors). In this calculation, the weights are the *squares* of the proportions falling into each tercile. The overall standard error is then the square root of this weighted average (Schafer and Kang 2008). The computations are:

$$Var = 0.30^2(1.212^2) + 0.30^2(1.074^2) + 0.40^2(0.904^2) = 0.367.$$

$$SE = \sqrt{0.367} = 0.606.$$

As DeMaris (2013) has suggested, *a test of the unintended pregnancy effect, adjusted for propensity scores*, is then accomplished with a t statistic. The degrees of freedom for t is taken to be the smallest error degrees of freedom from any of the individual ANCOVAs, which is 50 in this case. Hence, the test statistic for the effect of an unintended pregnancy, controlling for propensity scores, is $t = 1.76/0.606 = 2.904$, with a one-tailed p-value equal to 0.0027. As this is significant, we conclude, once again, that an unintended pregnancy elevates mothers' depression, controlling for pregnancy stress, and other covariates.

We have seen here that the propensity-score analysis essentially supports the conclusions from the analysis using ANCOVA. Frequently, researchers will double-check the robustness of their analyses by using other techniques that are designed to address potential pitfalls in the primary analysis. This process of double-checking one's results by performing multiple alternate analyses is referred to as *sensitivity analysis*, and is a staple of medical research.

Growth-Curve Modeling

In Chap. 8 we discussed survival analysis, in which the time until occurrence of a discrete event was the study endpoint. The discrete event in question was considered a change from one state (e.g., cancer free) to another (e.g., cancer recurrence). But what should we do if, rather than a discrete state, interest centers on the gradual change over time in a quantitative variable? The technique of choice in this case is variously referred to as *growth curve analysis* (GCA; e.g., Umberson et al. 2009) or the *linear mixed model* (Green et al. 2009). In this type of study, subjects are measured on more than one occasion, similar to the case of repeated measures ANOVA discussed in Chap. 6. The difference is that the primary explanatory variables are quantitative rather than qualitative. This necessitates more of a regression approach than an ANOVA strategy.

A simple example of the data scenario is illustrated in Fig. 9.2.

This figure depicts the *growth trajectories*, or patterns of growth, in a study endpoint (Y) over nine time periods (numbered 0–8) for five subjects. (Note that "growth" is a general term for change over time; the change may, in fact, be a decline rather than literally "growth" in the response.) Each subject shows a linear pattern of change over time. Most exhibit a linear increase in the study endpoint over time, although subject 3 shows a linear decrease. Each subject's growth in Y can be characterized by a linear regression equation with an intercept and a slope for Time. For example, subject 4 that shows the most pronounced positive growth (and is the top line in the figure) has equation:

$$Y_4 = 0.45 + 1.15\text{Time}.$$

Subject 3's growth in Y (represented by the bottom line in the figure) on the other hand has equation:

$$Y_3 = 0.35 - 0.15\text{Time}.$$

Fig. 9.2 Sample linear growth-curve trajectories for a study endpoint over time

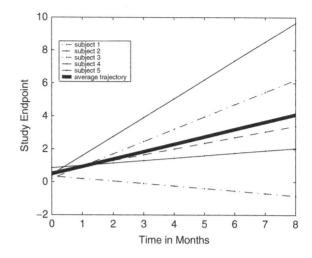

In general, any given subject's growth in Y can be represented by the equation:

$$Y_i = a_i + b_i \text{Time} + e_i, \tag{9.4}$$

where i denotes the ith subject, ranging from 1, 2, ... to n, and e_i represents the error term in the equation. In the simple example here, i ranges from 1 to 5 (and, to keep things simple, there are no errors in their regression equations). The i subscript on a and on b in (9.4) indicates that the intercept and slope of this equation vary from subject to subject, as is evident in Fig. 9.2. Because a and b vary over subjects, they are referred to as *random growth parameters* and are studied just like any other individual characteristics.

There are two principal aims in GCA (Singer and Willett 2003). The first is to describe the *average trajectory* in the study endpoint over time. This is the average of all the subjects' trajectories, which is found by simply averaging the intercepts and slopes of all subjects in the study. For the example here, the average intercept is 0.49 and the average slope is 0.45. The line representing the average intercept and slope is shown as the heavily shaded line in the middle of Fig. 9.2. The second aim is to understand *how subject characteristics affect variability around the average trajectory*. In other words, what explains the variability in individual subjects' intercepts and slopes? How are these affected by subjects' attributes?

Estimating the GCA Model

One way to understand how GCA is accomplished is to see it as consisting of two levels of analysis. First, it should be noted that the unit of analysis is not the individual subject, but rather the occasion of measurement for a given subject. That is, in the simple example above, there are nine occasions of measurement for each of five subjects, for a total of $9 \times 5 = 45$ units of analysis. We rewrite (9.4) to reflect this, using two subscripts for each unit of analysis: one for the subject (i) and one for the occasion of measurement (j).

$$Y_{ij} = a_i + b_i \text{Time}_j + e_{ij}. \qquad (9.5)$$

Equation (9.5) is the first-level equation that describes the nature of Time's effect on the study endpoint. Or, it describes the trajectory in the study endpoint over time. At the second level, the individual intercepts and slopes are themselves the study endpoints. They are modeled as being influenced by one or more subject character-istics. For example, suppose that one such characteristic is the subject's body-mass index (BMI):

$$\begin{aligned} a_i &= c + d\,\text{BMI}_i + u_i \\ b_i &= f + g\,\text{BMI}_i + w_i \end{aligned} \qquad (9.6)$$

At this level, we have two regression equations. One is for subjects' intercepts, and the other is for subjects' slopes. The terms u_i and w_i represent the error terms in *these* equations. Equations (9.5) and (9.6) can be combined into one composite equation. It is in this form, in fact, that it is represented in software packages such as SAS. If we simply substitute the mathematical definitions for a_i and b_i shown in (9.6) for the a_i and b_i in (9.5), we have the composite equation:

$$Y_{ij} = c + d\,\text{BMI}_i + f\,\text{Time}_j + g\,\text{BMI}_i * \text{Time}_j + (e_{ij} + u_i + w_i \text{Time}_j). \qquad (9.7)$$

Equation (9.7) shows a conventional regression equation for Y that includes main effects of both BMI and Time and an interaction between BMI and Time. Notice that BMI's effect on the intercept in (9.6) is shown in (9.7) as its effect on Y_{ij}. And BMI's effect on the slope in (9.6) is shown in (9.7) as an interaction between BMI and Time in their effects on Y_{ij}. That is, the effect of time—the linear trajectory itself—depends upon BMI, which is what Eqs. (9.6) are suggesting. We have col-lected all of the error terms as the parenthetical term in (9.7). This represents a much more complex error term than is found in linear regression estimated with ordinary least squares. The error term in (9.7) effectively models the complexity of the error that arises when the same subjects are measured multiple times on repeated occa-sions in a given study (Singer and Willett 2003). The Model shown in (9.7) is typi-cally estimated using maximum likelihood.

An Example: The Trajectory in Mother's Depression Over Time

In the NAPPS study mothers' depression was measured in all four waves. Therefore, we can examine the trajectory in depression over time, as well as the factors that affect that trajectory. To begin, we list the data records of the first four mothers in

Table 9.8 Listing of data lines for the first four mothers in the NAPPS study

Obs	subjid	time	unintend	m1pgst	moverben	modepr1	modepr2	modepr3	modepr4	depressn
1	1	0	0	8	2.12880	5	5	2	3.0000	5
2	1	4	0	8	2.12880	5	5	2	3.0000	5
3	1	7	0	8	2.12880	5	5	2	3.0000	2
4	1	13	0	8	2.12880	5	5	2	3.0000	3
5	2	0	0	11	2.06417	18	11	13	11.0000	18
6	2	4	0	11	2.06417	18	11	13	11.0000	11
7	2	7	0	11	2.06417	18	11	13	11.0000	13
8	2	13	0	11	2.06417	18	11	13	11.0000	11
9	3	0	0	5	3.39800	8	6	11	7.0000	8
10	3	4	0	5	3.39800	8	6	11	7.0000	6
11	3	7	0	5	3.39800	8	6	11	7.0000	11
12	3	13	0	5	3.39800	8	6	11	7.0000	7
13	4	0	0	5	−1.58919	7	1	3	2.0000	7
14	4	4	0	5	−1.58919	7	1	3	2.0000	1
15	4	7	0	5	−1.58919	7	1	3	2.0000	3
16	4	13	0	5	−1.58919	7	1	3	2.0000	2

the dataset. To accomplish the analysis, the data must be in *person-period* form. That is, there must be four data lines for each mother, one for each occasion of measurement. Each individual data line constitutes a unit of analysis for the study. Table 9.8 presents the data, as displayed by the software program SAS:

In this table, "Obs" is simply the number corresponding to each unit of analysis. "Subjid" is the subject identifier, which ranges here from 1 to 4. "Time" is in number of months since wave 1 and is coded 0, 4, 7, and 13. "Unintend" is the dummy variable for having an unintended pregnancy; all four mothers here had intended pregnancies. "M1pgst" is the pregnancy stressor index score. "Moverben" is the relative advantage score. "Modepr1–modepr4" are the depression scores for waves 1–4, respectively (used to create the time-varying depression score). "Depressn" is the time-varying depression score that is the study endpoint. We see that the factors measured at wave 1—unintend, m1pgst, and moverben—are simply duplicated on each of the four records for a given mother. These are referred to as *time-invariant* or *between-subjects* variables. On the other hand, Time and Depressn both vary in value over the four records for each mother. These are the *time-varying* or *within-subjects* variables in the study. The level 1 model utilizes the time-varying explanatory variables to predict the time-varying study endpoint. The level 2 model utilizes the time-invariant factors to predict the intercept and slope of the level 1 model. These principles were illustrated in (9.5, 9.6, and 9.7), above. Although there are 178 mothers in the study, a few cases are missing data at later time points. Hence, there are a total of 681 units of analysis in the study instead of $178 \times 4 = 712$. GCA is able to utilize all the available information even though some of the units of analysis have missing data (Fitzmaurice et al. 2004; Singer and Willett 2003).

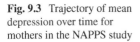

Fig. 9.3 Trajectory of mean depression over time for mothers in the NAPPS study

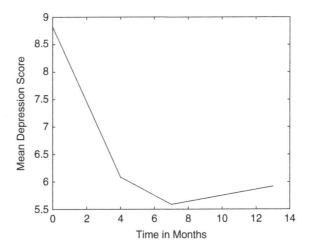

Table 9.9 Linear mixed model estimates for trajectory of mean depression over time for mothers in the NAPPS study

Explanatory variable	b	p-Value
Intercept	8.044	<0.0001
Time	−0.779	<0.0001
Time^2	0.044	<0.0001
Unintended pregnancy	1.555	0.0007
Number of pregnancy stressors	0.506	<0.0001
Time × number of pregnancy stressors	−0.077	0.0021
Time^2 × number of pregnancy stressors	0.006	0.0007
R^2	0.220	

Figure 9.3 shows the average trajectory in depression for the NAPPS mothers.

We see in this instance that the trajectory is not linear. It declines in a nonlinear fashion until about month 7, at which point it begins to rise again. How should we model this? It turns out that this type of pattern can be very effectively represented by including both Time and its square (i.e., Time^2) in the level 1 model. Models that include both X and X^2 are referred to as *quadratic* models. They will typically "fit" any type of curve characterized by just one bend, as in Fig. 9.3 (Singer and Willett 2003). Hence, the level 1 model has Time and Time^2 affecting mothers' depression. For the level 2 model, we will allow unintended pregnancy and the number of pregnancy stressors to affect the level-1 intercept. On the other hand, we will allow only the number of pregnancy stressors to affect the slopes of Time and Time^2. (The effect of an unintended pregnancy on these slopes was not significant.) This means that time will interact with pregnancy stress in its effect on mothers' depression. Or, the trajectory of mothers' depression over time will depend on how stressful their pregnancy was. In this analysis, only the level 1 intercept was specified as a random parameter, varying over subjects. There was not enough variability in the slopes of Time and Time^2 over subjects to also specify them as random parameters. Table 9.9 shows the results of estimating this GCA.

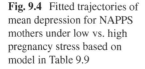

Fig. 9.4 Fitted trajectories of mean depression for NAPPS mothers under low vs. high pregnancy stress based on model in Table 9.9

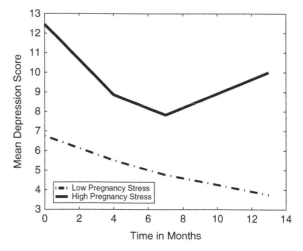

All factors in the model are quite significant, and the model accounts for about 22 % of the variance in mothers' depression over time. The intercept is the estimated average depression score at the initial survey (i.e., wave 1) for mothers with scores of 0 on all predictors. Hence, for mothers in wave 1 with intended pregnancies and no pregnancy stressors, average depression is estimated to be 8.044. The pattern over time is shown as a negative effect of Time and a positive effect of Time^2. This implies a negative linear trend that is becoming more and more positive over time. This is easily seen by examining the slope for Time for mothers reporting no pregnancy stressors. That slope is $-0.779 + 2(0.044)$ Time, which is $-0.779 + 0.088$ Time (the slope for the effect of X in $y = a + bX + cX^2$, by rules of calculus, is $b + 2cX$). That is, it is a function of Time itself. At Time 0 the slope is estimated to be $-0.779 + 0.088(0) = -0.779$. At Time 4, the slope is $-0.779 + 0.088(4) = -0.427$. At Time 8.85, the slope is $-0.779 + 0.088(8.85) = -0.0002$ (i.e., approximately zero). At Time 12, the slope is $-0.779 + 0.088(12) = 0.277$; and so forth. This nonlinear effect of time is indicating that the effect of passing time on mothers' average depression is curvilinear. At first, passing time diminishes depression, but this becomes a smaller and smaller effect over time. After sufficient time, there is once again an increase in depression with passing time. An unintended pregnancy is associated with an average depression score that is about 1.5 units higher at any given time, compared to the scores for mothers with intended pregnancies. Initially, the number of pregnancy stressors elevates average depression by about a half of a unit for each additional stressor. But it also significantly changes the trajectory in depression, since it interacts with both Time and Time^2.

To see this, regard Fig. 9.4. It compares the estimated trajectories in depression for two types of mothers, based on the model in Table 9.9. The first type has an unintended pregnancy and a pregnancy stressor index that is two standard deviations below the mean index score. These are referred to as the "low pregnancy stress" mothers. The second type has an unintended pregnancy but a pregnancy stressor index that is two standard deviations above the mean index score. These are the "high pregnancy stress" mothers.

The pattern shown is referred to as a *nonlinear interaction effect* (DeMaris 2004). This means that there is a different nonlinear trend in each group. It is clear that the trajectories take on different shapes, depending on the level of pregnancy stress. For low-stress mothers, there is an almost linear decline in depression over the follow-up period. But for high-stress mothers, the pattern is much more curvilinear. Depression declines in a nonlinear fashion to about month 7, and then begins a marked rise to the end of the follow-up period. Apparently, a stressful pregnancy has deleterious consequences for mothers' mental health even up to a year after the birth.

Fixed-Effects Regression Models

With the final technique discussed here, we come full circle and address an issue alluded to in Chap. 1. Recall the meat diet and PSA study in which we found that those on a meat diet had a higher average PSA level than those on a balanced diet. We noted that if men were not randomly assigned to each diet, then this finding could be confounded by a latent selection factor. Figure 9.5 shows the scenario, as depicted by Fig. 1.1:

The figure suggests, as noted in Chap. 1, that the positive "effect" of a meat diet on PSA level is completely caused by the negative association of a meat diet with health awareness and the negative effect of health awareness on PSA level. We further assume that health awareness is not measured in our study, so how can we control for it? It turns out that the influence of health awareness in the meat diet-PSA level association can be eliminated if a few conditions are satisfied. First, we have observations on men for at least two different points in time. Second, the level of a man's health awareness is a stable trait that does not change over time. Third, the *effect* of health awareness on PSA level is also stable and does not change over

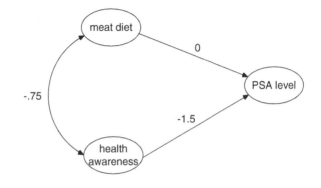

Fig. 9.5 Health awareness as an unmeasured confound in the meat diet-PSA level relationship (from Chap. 1)

time. If these conditions are met, health awareness can be controlled, *even though it is not measured*. It sounds like magic. But it's based on simple mathematics. Let HA_i be the health awareness level for the ith man and MD_{ij} be the dummy variable for being on a meat diet ($MD_{ij} = 1$) or not ($MD_{ij} = 0$) at a given time, j. The other condition that is required is that there be variation over time in men's diets. That is, a sufficient number of men have to switch diets over time from meat to balanced, or vice versa. Let PSA_{ij} be the ith man's PSA level at time j. PSA levels typically do fluctuate over time. Further, suppose we have two times on which men are observed, so that $j = 1$ and 2. Then we can write the equation for PSA level as a function of meat diet and health awareness at each time point:

$$PSA_{i1} = a_1 + bMD_{i1} + HA_i + e_{i1}, \tag{9.8}$$

$$PSA_{i2} = a_2 + bMD_{i2} + HA_i + e_{i2}. \tag{9.9}$$

Notice that the effect of a meat diet on PSA level, b, is presumed to be the same at each time point. This, however, is an assumption that can be tested (as we show below). It is also important to note that meat diet is *presumed to have a causal effect on PSA level*. Since they are both measured at the same time point at each observation period, the causal priority of meat diet cannot be established based on its chronological precedence. (Because a cause must precede an effect in time, were meat diet measured at an earlier time than PSA, its causal priority over PSA could be argued on that basis.) HA_i here is referred to as a *fixed effect*. A fixed effect is any unmeasured characteristic in our model that is correlated with one or more of the other predictors (Allison 2005, 2009; Wooldridge 2002). Notice also that HA_i has no j subscript because it does not change over time. Its effect, which is 1, is also the same at each time point, as per our required conditions. At this point, we simply subtract (9.8) from (9.9) to arrive at (9.10):

$$PSA_{i2} - PSA_{i1} = (a_2 - a_1) + b(MD_{i2} - MD_{i1}) + (e_{i2} - e_{i1}) \tag{9.10}$$

In this final equation, the fixed effect, HA_i, has been eliminated. We say that it has been "differenced away," and this differencing technique is referred to as the *first-differenced estimator* of the fixed-effects model (Wooldridge 2002). What is left in (9.10) is simply the effect of a meat diet, in the form of the effect of the *change* in meat-diet status over time (and it is obvious why meat-diet status must change over time for at least some men: otherwise this variable would equal zero for everyone). The response in (9.10) is similarly the *change* in PSA level over time. The intercept is the difference in intercepts between (9.9) and (9.8). But it is also the average change over time in PSA level, controlling for diet. The key to (9.10) is that the causal effect of meat diet on PSA level at each time, shown in (9.8) and (9.9), is the same b that is estimated by (9.10). Therefore, estimating (9.10) using ordinary least squares regression provides an unbiased estimate of that causal effect, *free from the influence of the unmeasured confound*.

An Example: Marital Conflict and Mothers' Depression

Once again, we draw on data from the NAPPS study to examine the effect of marital conflict on mothers' depression. Conflict between spouses is a stressor that appears to elevate depressive symptomatology, and more so in wives than husbands (DeMaris 2004). We presume at the outset that it is marital conflict that causes mothers' depression, and not the other way around. In NAPPS, the *marital conflict score* is the average of husbands' and wives' reports of the frequency of having both minor and major arguments. Each spouse's answer regarding each level of arguments is coded from 1 ("once a year or less") to 6 ("just about every day"). A higher score on the scale reflects more frequent arguments. Table 9.10 shows the effect of marital conflict on mothers' depression at the first and third waves of the study. These results are arrived at via linear regression models run separately for each wave of data. An unintended pregnancy and the pregnancy stressor index are included in the models as control variables.

To begin, the intercept for the wave 1 regression is substantially higher than the intercept for wave 3. This suggests that, net of other factors, average depression is higher at wave 1, during the third trimester of pregnancy. Marital conflict indeed has the expected significant positive effect on mothers' depression, controlling for an unintended pregnancy and pregnancy stress. Each unit increase in marital conflict raises average depression by anywhere from a half to almost two-thirds of a unit. As before, both an unintended pregnancy and pregnancy stress also add significantly to the depression level. Although these findings make substantive sense, it is unclear whether the coefficient for marital conflict represents a causal effect. Could it be simply that poorer-quality marriages are characterized by greater conflict and also lead to higher levels of the wife's depression? Figure 9.6 depicts this alternative scenario:

This model suggests that the positive relationship between conflict and depression is being driven by unmeasured marital distress. That is, marital distress is associated with greater conflict and, at the same time, precipitates greater depression in wives. It is entirely possible that once marital distress is controlled, conflict has no effect on depression. For this reason, the path from conflict to depression is shown with a question mark.

Table 9.10 Cross-sectional regression models for the effect of marital conflict on mothers' depression

Explanatory variable	Wave 1		Wave 3	
	b	p-Value	b	p-Value
Intercept	5.247	<0.0001	1.287	0.1516
Marital conflict[a]	0.489	0.0022	0.621	<0.0001
Unintended pregnancy[b]	1.544	0.0083	1.561	0.0035
Number of pregnancy stressors[b]	0.451	<0.0001	0.286	0.0026

[a]Measured in each wave
[b]Measured in wave 1, only

Fig. 9.6 Diagram of marital distress as a Fixed Effect Confounding the Marital Conflict-depression Association

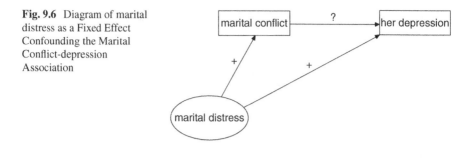

Table 9.11 Fixed-effects regression via the first-differenced estimator for the effect of marital conflict on mothers' depression

Explanatory variable	b	p-Value
Intercept	−3.195	<0.0001
Difference in marital conflict[a]	0.411	0.0421
Unintended pregnancy[b]	0.017	0.9757
Number of pregnancy stressors[b]	−0.150	0.1268

[a]Measured as wave 3 conflict–wave 1 conflict
[b]Measured in wave 1, only

Table 9.11 presents the fixed-effects regression analysis results. The change in mothers' depression from wave 1 to wave 3 is regressed on the change in marital conflict from wave 1 to wave 3, along with the two control variables.

Once again, we regard the intercept first. It suggests that, net of other factors, there is an average drop of about 3 units in mothers' depression over time. We see that the effect of marital conflict has been reduced slightly, but is still significant ($p = 0.0421$) and positive. The results suggest that, controlling for an unintended pregnancy and pregnancy stress, each unit increase in conflict adds about four-tenths of a unit to average depression. Thus, it appears that the effect of conflict is not just an artifact of its correlation with an underlying stable characteristic of the couples that also affects depression. This finding lends support to the proposition that marital conflict elevates mothers' depression level. Nevertheless, there is a caveat: this analysis only controls for unmeasured couple (or mother) characteristics that are stable over time and have stable effects on depression. Should there be an unmeasured characteristic that does not exhibit these conditions, it could still be driving the results.

We notice that the two control variables are very nonsignificant, despite both being very significant in the separate regressions by study wave. In fact, the presence of time-invariant controls such as these in the model is not necessary. Just as the differencing of (9.9) and (9.8) eliminated any stable unmeasured confound, it also eliminates time-invariant factors that have unchanging effects on the response. Since both unintended pregnancy and pregnancy stress were measured in wave 1, they necessarily exhibit no change in value at wave 3. Also, as long as they have the same effect on wave 3 depression as on wave 1 depression, they both have stable effects on the response. Therefore, they are differenced away by the subtraction that produced (9.10) in the same way that HA_i was eliminated. Nevertheless, they are controlled for, just as HA_i is controlled in this analysis. However, if their effects on conflict were different in wave 3 compared to wave 1, then they would not be differenced away and they would appear in (9.10). In that scenario, the effect of each control on depression would be different, depending on the time of measurement of depression. Or, each control would interact with Time in its effect on depression. Including the two controls in (9.10) is therefore a way of testing whether such interactions obtain. The results shown in Table 9.11 indicate that there are no such interaction effects. In other words, the assumption that these two control variables have invariant effects on depression over time appears to be supported. Whether the effect of conflict on depression is the same at each time point—an assumption of fixed-effects regression—can also be easily tested. One simply includes wave 1 conflict in (9.10), along with the change in conflict. A test for the significance of the coefficient of wave 1 conflict in that equation is a test for the change in the effect of conflict across time periods (Allison 2005). When that was performed (not shown), it turned out to be nonsignificant. Hence, there is no evidence to suggest that the effect of conflict on depression is different at each time period. As a final comment, fixed-effects regression analysis is not the only technique for controlling an unobserved confound. However, the complexity of other techniques renders them somewhat beyond the scope of the present primer (see, e.g., DeMaris 2012, for two other such techniques).

Applications

In this section of the chapter, we illustrate several applications of the aforementioned techniques that have appeared in the medical literature in recent years.

Poisson Regression

We have already discussed the study by Rosenfeld and colleagues (2012) above. Here, we revisit that study and consider its results. Cystic Fibrosis (CF) is a debilitating and potentially fatal illness with particularly pernicious consequences for young children. The authors note the primary difficulty engendered by the disease (p. 2269):

> Dysfunctional ion transport leads to reduced airway surface liquid volume in CF and reduction in mucociliary clearance. Retained mucus serves as a nidus for chronic infection and exaggerated, sustained neutrophilic inflammation, resulting in progressive air- way obstruction and bronchiectasis. Hypertonic saline has been demonstrated to increase airway surface liquid in bronchial epithelial cells in vitro and to improve defective mucociliary clearance in patients with CF.

To examine the efficacy and safety of hypertonic saline inhalation in patients under 6 years old with CF, the authors conducted a 30-center randomized clinical trial. Children aged 4–60 months with a confirmed diagnosis of CF were randomly assigned to inhale either 7 % hypertonic saline (treatment group) or 0.9 % isotonic saline (control group) twice daily for 48 weeks. The primary outcome was the number of pulmonary exacerbations over the observation period of up to 48 weeks (some children were not observed for this entire follow-up period). The authors couch the study endpoint as (p. 2270) the "rate of pulmonary exacerbations," since they control for the observation time for each child as an offset. In their own words (pp. 2271–2272):

> The primary outcome, pulmonary exacerbation rate, was compared between groups accord-
> ing to intent-to treat principles using a Poisson log-linear regression model with the log of
> observation time as an offset. Observation time was defined as time since randomization to
> last in-clinic visit or follow-up telephone call. (One participant's observation time was
> defined to be one-half day, because he or she did not have an in-clinic visit or follow-up
> telephone call after randomization.) The rate ratio was also analyzed with adjustment for
> age category and site.

The authors refer to the model as a "log-linear" regression because, as we saw above, the log of the mean count is the response variable. And this is modeled as a linear function, or formula, involving the independent variables. We see that obser-vation time, which was the number of weeks that the children were under observa-tion in the study, was used as the offset here. The authors describe the dependent variable in the last sentence as the "rate ratio," because, again as we have seen above, using an offset implies that one is studying the *rate* of event occurrence. Age category, coded as less than 30 months vs. 30 months or more, and site were employed as covariates in the model.

Ultimately, the authors found no significant effect on the exacerbation rate for treatment with hypertonic saline, as opposed to the control condition. They detail their results in the following passage (p. 2273):

> The pulmonary exacerbation rate was 2.3 (95% CI, 2.0-2.5) per person-year among partici-
> pants randomized to receive hypertonic saline and 2.3 (95% CI, 2.1-2.6) per person-year
> among participants randomized to receive isotonic saline. The ratio of the mean pulmonary
> exacerbation rate in the hypertonic saline group compared with the isotonic saline group
> was 0.97 (95% CI, 0.83-1.13).

The pulmonary exacerbation rate is couched in terms of person-years in each study group. Children, on the other hand, were followed for at most 48 weeks—not quite a year. No matter. It is a simple matter to convert the exacerbation rate over 48 weeks to 1 that is over a year by multiplying it by the ratio 48/52. So suppose the average number of exacerbations in, say, the hypertonic saline group was 119.6. It turns out that mean duration of study participation for this group was 47 weeks (Rosenfeld et al. 2012). So the average exacerbation rate in this group was $119.6/47 = 2.545$ per 47-week period. Converted to a 52-week period, the rate is $2.545 (47/52) = 2.3$. Notice that the authors refer to "the ratio of the mean pulmonary exacerbation rate" for treatment vs. control groups. This is simply the exponentiated coefficient for the treatment effect. That is, the effect of treatment with hypertonic saline in the Poisson regression model was −0.03. Therefore, the multiplicative impact of treatment on the mean exacerbation rate, itself, was then $\exp(-0.03) = 0.97$. As the 95 % confidence interval for this effect contains 1, indicating no effect, this effect is clearly nonsignificant.

Propensity-Score Analysis and Multiple Imputation

Wahbi and colleagues (2012) conducted a retrospective study of patients suffering from Steinert disease, also known as myotonic dystrophy type I (DM1). According to the authors, DM1 is the most common inherited neuromuscular disease in adults. Up to one-third of patients with DM1 succumb to sudden death due to progression of conduction-system disease leading to complete atrioventricular block (Wahbi et al. 2012). The objective of the study was to assess the difference in survival rates for patients treated with an invasive, vs. a noninvasive, strategy for this disease. The authors retrospectively identified 914 consecutive patients over the age of 18 from a French hospital who were admitted between January 2000 and December 2009 for management of DM1. Patients were divided into two groups based on their treatment. The invasive strategy group consisted of all patients undergoing a systematic electrophysiological study followed by the implanting of a pacing device. The noninvasive strategy group included patients who underwent neither of these treatments, but were simply subjected to regular surveillance. The principal endpoint of the study was the overall survival probability. Survival analysis was conducted with the Cox proportional hazards model, with adjustment for potential confounding covariates. The authors employed propensity-score adjustments to these analyses. In the following passage, they explain their reasoning (p. 1294):

> Because this was an observational study, a propensity score–based approach was used to limit the biases of between-group comparisons. The propensity score is the probability that a patient with specific baseline characteristics would receive an experimental intervention (in this case, the invasive strategy). Two patients with identical propensity scores included in the invasive strategy group and in the noninvasive strategy group could be considered randomly assigned to each group, and conditioning on the propensity score theoretically leads to unbiased estimates of between-group differences. We computed the propensity score using logistic regression, in which the comparison between the invasive strategy group and the noninvasive strategy group was the dependent variable and the baseline characteristics were the independent variables.

The propensity scores were incorporated into the Cox regression in a number of alternate ways, following the principle of conducting a sensitivity analysis. For example, in one analysis, they were divided into quintiles and these were employed as covariates in the model, with or without other covariates. In another analysis, the raw propensity score was employed in the model as a quantitative covariate. In yet a third strategy, patients were matched on their propensity scores, and the Cox model was run with adjustment for the correlation "within matched sets" (p. 1298).

The authors also resorted to replacing missing data with multiple imputation. As they explain (pp. 1294–1295):

> The missing data on vital capacity for 60 patients, size of CTG amplification for 38 patients, left ventricular ejection fraction for 11 patients, PR interval for 10 patients, and QRS duration for 5 patients were handled through multiple imputations using the chained equations method, taking into account the baseline mortality hazard. The 30 independent, imputed data sets that were generated were analyzed separately. Estimates of the model variables were then pooled over the 30 imputations (according to the rule by Rubin and Schenker) to present single estimates and standard errors for each variable.

In this particular case, the authors generated 30 different imputed datasets and then combined the Cox estimates from all 30 analyses into one set of estimates and standard errors. The "chained equations method" is a particular estimation technique for arriving at the imputed values.

Ultimately, all analyses showed a distinct advantage of the invasive treatment over the noninvasive strategy. Hazard ratios for the overall hazard of death favored the invasive-strategy group and ranged from 0.47 to 0.61, depending on how propensity scores were incorporated into the analysis. As the authors acknowledge (1298), this translates into an 11.3–16.9 % higher probability of survival at 9 years that is associated with the invasive strategy. The hazard of sudden death was also 75 % lower in the invasive-strategy group, compared to the noninvasive-strategy group.

Growth-Curve Analysis I

Hewitt and Turrell (2011) investigated the consequences for psychological and physical health of marital separation. They theorized that the spouse who initiated the separation would have more feelings of control over the process. This increased control would then serve to mitigate the negative consequences of the marital disruption. They therefore hypothesized that (a) those who separate would have worse physical and mental health than those who remained married, and (b) among the separators, the initiators would fare better than others. Their data came from a longitudinal Australian population survey in which a sample of 1,786 men and 2,068 women in their first marriages were followed from 2001 to 2007. There were seven waves of the survey conducted at yearly intervals. Their primary explanatory variable, marital status, was coded into four categories: stable marriage, self-initiated separation, partner-initiated separation, and jointly initiated separation. Eight dimensions of physical and mental health constituted the study endpoints. These were all derived from a set of items referred to as the SF-36 on the survey questionnaire. One such outcome was referred to as "general health (overall personal health)" (Hewitt and Turrell 2011, p. 1310).

The analytic technique the authors employed was a growth-curve approach with only the intercept in the equation as a random growth parameter (as in our NAPPS example, above). Other nuances of their strategy can be seen in the authors' description of their statistical model (pp. 1310–1311):

> Changes in physical and mental health with marital separation were examined using a series of linear random intercept models. This modeling approach accounts for the clustering of observations within persons and has the capacity to handle unbalanced panel designs (inconsistent numbers of observations per person)...Secondly, we included 1-year lag measures for health in each of the models of the 8 dimensions of the SF-36. The lagged health measures indicated the participant's health status in the previous wave, which allowed us to take into account the effect of prior health status on current health status. This also helped us control for unobserved heterogeneity between individuals and reduced the potential for reverse causality (i.e., the possibility that poor health caused the marital transition).

The technique is described as a "linear random intercept" model, i.e., a linear mixed model with just the intercept as a random growth parameter. This model is described as allowing for the "clustering of observations within persons." This refers to the fact that people are repeatedly surveyed over time. Therefore, each person is contributing seven observations, or cases, to the dataset. Since these are all from the same person, they are said to be "clustered" within the person. This situation creates a more complicated equation error that is nicely accommodated using linear mixed modeling. The design is said to be "unbalanced," due to the fact that some years of data are missing for some of the participants. Therefore, not everyone is contributing the same number of observations to the dataset. Finally, including the 1-year lagged version of the health measure in the analysis of any given health measure is described as assisting in the control for "unobserved heterogeneity." This term refers to an unobserved, or unmeasured, confounding variable that could skew results. A model that includes a lagged version of Y as an explanatory variable is referred to as an *autoregressive model*, and also helps to control for reverse causation. With this approach, the effects of other explanatory variables can be shown to be the effects on the *change* in Y over time. This provides some assurance that it is not simply the case that unhealthier people at any given time are more prone to separation than others and are also unhealthier than others at a subsequent time period.

The authors' hypotheses were generally confirmed. For example, Fig. 9.7 (Figure 4 in the article) depicts the change over time in general health for women respondents:

The authors' description of these results is (p. 1312): "Women whose partner initiated separation had significantly lower levels of general health (−5.39) than women who self-initiated separation, and this gap widened over time (Figure 4)." This pattern is evident in the figure: The dash-dot line, representing partner-initiated separation, begins to fall below the solid line, representing self-initiated separation, in the year before the separation. And this gap grows ever wider over time. Curiously, the general health of those who either self- or jointly initiated the separation becomes increasingly better than that of the stably married women over time. However, this gap may not be significant, as the authors do not highlight this finding. Although the figure is not shown, findings were similar for men (p. 1312): "...men who self-initiated separation had improved general health in comparison with stably married men (4.85). Men whose partner initiated separation had significantly worse general health than men who self-initiated separation (−5.28)."

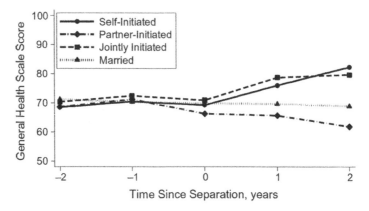

Fig. 9.7 Predicted mean Short Form 36 general health scores for women who separated (self-initiated, partner-initiated, and jointly initiated) relative to those who remained married, HILDA Survey, waves 1–7 (2001–2007). HILDA, Households, Income and Labour Dynamics in Australia. Reprinted with permission of Oxford University Press from Hewitt and Turrell (2011)

Growth-Curve Analysis II

Another example of the linear mixed model comes from the work by Green and associates (2009). Their interest was in assessing the efficacy of tarenflurbil to slow the rate of cognitive decline in patients with mild Alzheimer disease (AD). Tarenflurbil is a selective Amyloid-β peptide ($A\beta_{42}$) lowering agent. As the authors note (p. 2557), "In mouse models of AD, tarenflurbil prevents learning and memory deficits and reduces $A\beta_{42}$ brain concentrations." The authors conducted a randomized, double-blind study to compare tarenflurbil with placebo for 18 months at 133 participating trial sites. The sample consisted of patients with mild AD severity and included 809 in the placebo group vs. 840 in the tarenflurbil group. The latter received 800 mg of the drug twice daily (Green et al. 2009). The authors describe the primary study endpoints 2558:

> Co-primary efficacy outcomes were cognition as assessed by the Alzheimer Disease Assessment Scale–Cognitive Subscale (ADAS-Cog, 80- point version) and functional ability as assessed by the Alzheimer Disease Cooperative Study activities of daily living (ADCS-ADL, 78-point scale).

Although not articulated in this chapter, higher scores on the ADAS-Cog reflect a *decline* in cognitive ability. Lower scores on the ADCS-ADL, on the other hand, indicate a decline in activities of daily living.

In the following passage (p. 2559), the authors detail their statistical strategy, a combination of ANCOVA with the linear mixed model:

> The primary analysis was performed on changes from baseline to month 18 in total score for ADAS-Cog and ADCS-ADL. Slopes of total scores for both scales were evaluated as a secondary outcome…. Change-from-baseline analyses were conducted using an analysis of covariance model with treatment group, clinical site, and current use of acetylcholinesterase inhibitor, memantine, or both as fixed effects with the baseline score as the covariate.

The slopes analyses were conducted using a repeated measures linear mixed model, with random intercepts and slopes, baseline score and time as covariates, factors for treatment group, clinical site, and current use of acetylcholinesterase inhibitor, memantine, or both, and a term for treatment group x time interaction. Time was treated as a continuous variable.

Let's "deconstruct" this description. The first analytic technique mentioned was an ANCOVA in which the outcome—ADAS-Cog, say—was regressed on treatment group, baseline ADAS-Cog, and covariates. The effect of treatment in such a model is synonymous with its effect on the *change in the outcome from baseline*. For example, the change that comes closest to being significant was the change from baseline to month 15 (Table 2, p. 2562): 5.91 for the tarenflurbil group vs. 5.11 for placebo ($p = 0.097$). In this instance, the tarenflurbil group showed more of a cognitive decline at month 15, but the difference was not significant.

The second technique is described as a "repeated measures linear mixed model," i.e., a linear mixed model. Using the term "repeated measures" stresses that it is a growth-curve model, since the linear mixed model has other applications. Any situation involving units of analysis that are clustered within larger units is appropriate for this type of model. So this model could be used if we studied families (different family members are clustered within each family), schools (different children are clustered within each school), and so on (Raudenbush and Bryk 2002). In this model, as well, the baseline outcome is included as a covariate. Time in months was employed as the time factor, and the intercept and slope of the effect of time are both specified as random growth parameters. Moreover, an interaction is allowed between treatment group and time, similar to the interaction of number of pregnancy stressors and time in the NAPPS example above (see Table 9.9 and Fig. 9.4). From Table 2 of the study (p. 2562), the slope of the effect of time on the ADAS-Cog was 5.22 for tarenflurbil and 5.06 for placebo ($p = 0.69$). The slope of time's effect on the ADCS-ADL was -7.12 for tarenblurbil and -7.08 for placebo ($p = 0.95$). These results were disappointing. As the authors noted (pp. 2561–2562): "Tarenflurbil did not slow cognitive decline or loss of ADLs in patients with mild AD nor did any secondary outcome measure or post hoc analysis favor tarenflurbil."

Fixed-Effects Regression

A nicely articulated example of the fixed-effects regression model comes from the article by Duncan and Rees (2005). The authors were interested in reevaluating the potential causal effect of cigarette smoking on depressive symptomatology. Although a strong association between the two had been shown in prior studies, the authors argue that the association may not be causal. They suggest that an underlying environmental or genetic factor could predispose individuals to both smoking and depression. The point of the study, in their words, was (p. 461):

In order to explore the role played by difficult-to-measure environmental and genetic influences potentially correlated with both smoking and depression, we compare estimates from standard regression models, which can be thought of as providing "naïve" estimates of the effect of smoking on depression, with fixed effects estimates that completely control for time-invariant factors.

That is, the authors propose to compare ordinary least squares regression estimates (i.e., standard linear-regression results) of the effect of smoking on depression, with those from fixed-effects regression models. As outlined above, the latter control for any time-invariant attribute having a time-invariant effect on depression that might be responsible for the smoking-depression association.

The authors use data from the National Longitudinal Study of Adolescent Health. This is a stratified random sample of students in all high schools with more than 30 students in the USA. Wave 1 of the study was conducted in 1995; the same students were resurveyed approximately a year later (wave 2). A total of 13,068 students were in the analysis, 6,320 males and 6,748 females. Smoking status was captured with two variables: a dummy variable for whether the student was a smoker at each wave, and the number of packs per month smoked. Depressive symptomatology was measured with the aforementioned CES-D; the authors employed 18 of the total 20 items originally included in the scale. In the following passage (pp. 462, 464), the authors explain the advantage of the fixed-effects approach (where π_1 and π_2 represent the effects on depressive symptomatology in wave 2 of, respectively, being a smoker and the number of packs smoked per month, each assessed in wave 1):

> Estimating equation 1 using ordinary least squares will produce unbiased estimates of π_1 and π_2 if the error term, $\varepsilon_{i,\ t=2}$, is uncorrelated with smoking behavior. However, if unobservable environmental or genetic factors are correlated with both the CES-D score at follow-up and smoking behavior, then ordinary least squares estimates will be biased. Furthermore, because the baseline CES-D score is not included as an explanatory variable in equation 1, this approach is subject to a problem of reverse causality: That is, if preexisting depression leads to smoking at baseline, then it is inappropriate to interpret ordinary least squares estimates of π_1 and π_2 as the effect of smoking on depressive symptomatology. We address these problems by taking fuller advantage of the longitudinal nature of the Adolescent Health data by modifying equation 1 to include individual-specific intercepts, often called "fixed effects."

The findings from the ordinary least squares regression are shown in Table 9.12 (only the smoking variables and four of the six baseline (i.e., wave 1) controls are shown):

Here, it is clear that being a smoker at baseline is significantly (since the 95 % CI does not contain zero) associated with higher depressive symptomatology for both males and females. We see that the number of monthly packs smoked is associated with higher depressive symptomatology for females, but not males. Of the controls, having a disability, being older (vs. being 11–13 years old), being Black, being Hispanic, being of an "other" race/ethnicity, receiving welfare (for males), and having an alcoholic parent (for females) are all associated with greater depressive symptomatology.

Table 9.13 presents the fixed-effects regression results:

We see in the table footnote that each student contributes two observations to the study: their data from wave 1 and their data from wave 2. Thus, the sample sizes for males and females are double what they were in the linear regression analysis (i.e., $6,320 \times 2 = 12,640$ and $6,748 \times 2 = 13,496$). The comment about age refers to the fact that the time interval between waves 1 and 2 was not exactly the same for each student. If it were, then the differencing process that eliminates the fixed effects would include the difference *wave 2 age–wave 1 age* in the model. However, this would be

Table 9.12 Ordinary least squares regression results showing the effect of baseline smoking on the Center for Epidemiologic Studies Depression Score at Follow-up, by Gender, National Longitudinal Study of Adolescent Health, 1995–1996 [Reprinted with permission of Oxford University Press from Duncan and Rees (2005)]

	Males		Females	
	Marginal effect (increased score)	95 % confidence interval†	Marginal effect (increased score)	95 % confidence interval†
Smoker at baseline	2.85	2.01, 3.68	2.92	2.14, 3.71
Packs per month at baseline	0.06	–0.046, 0.057	0.06	0.0004, 0.116
Baseline controls Disability	3.03	1.26, 4.81	3.97	1.55, 6.38
Age (years)				
14–15	1.55	0.85, 2.24	1.70	1.07, 2.32
16–17	1.67	0.91, 2.43	1.52	0.90, 2.13
$\geq$18	3.17	2.03, 4.32	1.87	0.52, 3.23
Race/ethnicity variables				
Black	1.88	1.14, 2.63	2.00	1.12, 2.87
Other	1.52	0.55, 2.49	1.87	0.82, 2.92
Hispanic	0.93	0.06, 1.79	1.59	0.43, 2.75
Household variables				
Two-parent home	0.11	–0.57, 0.79	–0.29	–0.92, 0.33
Welfare receipt	1.20	0.33, 2.08	0.88	–0.33, 2.09
Alcoholic parent	0.11	–0.64, 0.85	1.16	0.38, 1.93

Table 9.13 Fixed-effects regression results from the Duncan and Rees Study. Reprinted with permission of Oxford University Press from Duncan and Rees (2005)

	Males		Females	
	Marginal effect (increased score)	95 % confidence interval	Marginal effect (increased score)	95 % confidence interval
Smoker	0.66	0.28, 1.04	1.16	0.69, 1.63
Packs per month	0.019	–0.004, 0.043	0.01	–0.02, 0.05
Age	–0.14	–0.32, 0.04	–0.32	–0.52, –0.11
F statistic	6.00		10.18	
p Value	<0.001		<0.001	
Sample size (no.)	12,640		13,496	

Each respondent contributes two observations to the estimation of this model (one from the baseline survey and the other from the follow-up survey). As a consequence, both the baseline and follow-up Center for Epidemiologic Studies Depression scores are utilized in the estimation of the parameters. Age is not captured by the individual fixed effects, because the time between the baseline and follow-up interviews was not uniform across respondents. All other baseline control variables are absorbed by the individual fixed effects

the same constant for every student. For example, if there were exactly 12 months in between waves for every student, then the age difference would be 12 for everyone. A variable like this that exhibits no variability among respondents would be automatically excluded from the regression. That age can be included here is due to the varying follow-up time intervals for students. The phrase "All other baseline control variables are absorbed by the individual fixed effects" is statistical jargon for the fact that the differencing process that eliminates the fixed effects also eliminates all other time-invariant controls (assuming they have time-invariant effects on depressive symptomatology). Nevertheless, all these factors are controlled in the fixed-effects analysis. Notice now that the effect of smoking status, although still significant for both genders, is dramatically reduced, compared to the linear regression results. And the number of packs smoked is no longer significant for either gender. As the authors note (p. 468), "…controlling for unobservable factors dramatically reduces the estimated effect of smoking…These estimates suggest that smoking has, at most, an extremely modest impact on depressive symptomatology."

Conclusion: Looking Back, Looking Forward

Looking Back

At this point, we have completed our statistical journey. In this primer, we have examined a range of techniques that are central to the statistical enterprise. We began by considering an issue that is at the heart of science: estimating causal effects. We then set out to understand the fundamental tools of statistics that enable us to accomplish this task: describing the center and spread of a variable's distribution, describing population distributions, coming to grips with the sampling distribution of a statistic—arguably the most important single concept in inferential statistics. We then considered the twin inferential goals of estimation of population parameters and testing hypotheses about population parameters. In the process, we briefly entertained the issue of the power of a statistical test. Next we investigated various means of testing the association between two variables, depending upon how each was measured. This was followed by an excursion into linear regression modeling, introducing the very important enterprise of the statistical modeling of a study endpoint. Continuing the modeling theme, we examined a number of different modeling techniques that were tailored to the particular manner in which the dependent variable was measured. These included multiple linear regression, repeated-measures ANOVA, logistic regression, survival analysis, Poisson and negative binomial regression, and linear mixed modeling. Along the way, we have considered additional techniques designed to handle particular problems in statistics, such as multiple imputation, propensity-score analysis, and fixed-effects regression models. By now it is hoped that the reader has a good understanding of the purpose and meaning of the statistical procedures that he or she is likely to encounter in the medical literature.

Looking Forward

Statistics is an ever-evolving science: New statistical procedures are being invented on a daily basis. It is therefore impossible for any single book to cover all of the techniques the reader is likely to encounter, let alone all of the new tools that will come along after that book is in print. Therefore, we outline here a prescription for understanding foreign statistical concepts and tools that the reader may encounter in the future. All statistical procedures are designed to aid in the scientific enterprise of determining the causes of real-world phenomena. Toward this end, the statistician uses different tools to accomplish a variety of goals:

Describe Data. We have discussed only a few of the many ways in which statisticians describe variable distributions, focusing on the mean, median, percentile, variance, and standard deviation. We have also seen a few graphical techniques for depicting distributions, such as the histogram and bar chart. There are many other such tools that we have not discussed. And in all likelihood, new techniques for this purpose will be available in the future. It should be readily apparent when the user is being presented with statistical or graphical summaries of variable distributions.

Estimate Parameters. Confidence intervals are the primary means of presenting estimates of population parameters. We have also mentioned some of the techniques that statisticians use to estimate parameters, particularly in statistical models. Such techniques include least squares and maximum likelihood estimation. However, there are many other such procedures not covered here, such as method of moments estimation, generalized least squares, partial least squares, and so forth. New procedures for parameter estimation are likely to evolve as time goes on; the reader should be on the lookout for these.

Model a Study Endpoint. We have seen that a statistical model is a set of one or more equations that describe how the study endpoint was "generated" in the population. The model always includes a set of assumptions to go along with the equations; if those assumptions are satisfied, the model may produce useful estimates of predictor effects. If one or more of those assumptions is violated, the estimates of predictor effects may be invalid, or, at worst, utter nonsense. Most statistical models are a variant of the linear regression model, as we have seen. There is an equation relating the study endpoint to a set of explanatory variables. In this primer, we have considered only *single-equation models* or models consisting of only one equation for the study endpoint. There are many techniques that simultaneously employ more than one equation to describe a study endpoint. Examples are *instrumental-variables regression,* the *nonrecursive model*, and the *sample-selection model*. And there are other techniques that employ multiple equations to simultaneously model a set of related study endpoints. Examples of this are *path analysis, factor analysis*, and *seemingly unrelated regression models*. These are rarely used in medicine and so have not been covered in this primer. Regardless, the reader will be able to recognize when a model is being used to describe one or more study endpoints. And regardless of how arcane the technique, interest will be centered on the effects of one or more predictors on the study endpoint. These are relatively straightforward to decipher.

Estimate a Causal Effect. We have seen that causal effects can be estimated in an unbiased fashion when subjects are randomly assigned to treatment conditions. Since many "treatments" of interest cannot be randomly assigned, however, we must resort to statistical legerdemain to deal with potential biases that may arise. We have considered some of these tools, in particular, statistical control, propensity-score analysis, and fixed-effects regression modeling. There are other procedures that have not been covered here, e.g., *instrumental-variables regression* or the *Heckman self-selection model* (DeMaris 2012). Regardless, the reader should be aware that, with nonexperimental data, researchers will typically try to employ statistical adjustments of some kind to eliminate the threat of unobserved heterogeneity (or a latent confound).

Adjust for Measurement Error. Ideally, all study endpoints and predictor variables are exactly measured and all subjects provide complete data on them. In practice, this is rarely the case. Missing data are a perennial problem. We have seen that multiple imputation is a state-of-the-art technique for replacing missing data. New, improved procedures for this purpose are likely to come along in the future. Although most medical conditions and treatments are often exactly measured, some variables of particular interest are more subjectively assessed. Examples are quality of life or depressive symptomatology. There can be considerable measurement error in such variables, which, in turn, limits our ability to estimate how they are affected by explanatory variables (Bollen 1989). Statisticians are always on the lookout for improved measurement techniques. One statistical development, which has seen little application so far in medical journals, is *structural equation modeling* (Bollen 1989). This statistical apparatus allows data analysts to account for measurement error in variables and thereby achieve more accurate estimates of predictor effects on a study endpoint. We can expect many more imaginative approaches to this problem to come along in the future.

In sum, the topics covered in this primer provide the fundamentals needed for understanding statistics as employed in medicine today. They also lay the groundwork for coming to terms with new techniques that readers are likely to encounter as statistical applications in medicine continue to evolve. Hence, the reader should go forward with confidence, trusting that he or she has the statistical background to be a knowledgeable consumer of this elegant and powerful craft.

Glossary of Statistical Terms

Accelerated failure-time model: A type of regression model in survival analysis in which the study endpoint is the natural logarithm of survival time; it necessitates knowledge of the probability distribution for survival time, because the estimation method is maximum likelihood.

Adjusted means: Estimated means on a study endpoint for different groups after controlling for the groups' different distributions on the quantitative control variables in an ANCOVA model.

Adjusted R^2: A version of R^2 with the property that, unlike R^2, it can decline as new predictors are added to a regression model. The adjusted R^2 is better than R^2 as an estimator of the R^2 for the population model.

Alpha reliability (a.k.a. Cronbach's alpha): A measure ranging from 0 to 1 that represents the proportion of a composite measure (i.e., a sum of individual items) that consists of a stable underlying attribute.

Alpha-level for a test: The criterion probability that is compared to the p value to determine whether the null hypothesis is to be rejected or not. The usual alpha level is 0.05.

Analysis of covariance (ANCOVA): A variation on linear regression in which quantitative explanatory variables are combined with qualitative explanatory variables in a regression model.

Analysis of variance (ANOVA): A type of bivariate or multivariable statistical analysis for a quantitative study endpoint when all explanatory variables are qualitative in measurement.

Area under the curve or AUC (a.k.a. concordance index): In logistic regression, the area under the ROC curve; it represents the likelihood that a case will have a higher predicted probability of the event than a control across the range of criterion

A. DeMaris and S.H. Selman, *Converting Data into Evidence: A Statistics Primer for the Medical Practitioner*, DOI 10.1007/978-1-4614-7792-1,
© Springer Science+Business Media New York 2013

probabilities. In Cox regression, it's referred to as the concordance, or *"c"* index and serves the comparable function of indicating the predictive power of the model.

Association: A relationship between two variables in which the distribution of the first variable changes over the levels of the second variable. That is, the second variable appears to influence the distribution on the first variable. If the second variable causes the first, then the two variables should be associated.

Autoregressive model: A regression model in which one of the explanatory variables is an earlier measurement of the study endpoint.

Average causal effect: The average of the causal effects for all cases in the population.

Bar graph: A graphical display of a variable's distribution, in which the heights of bars represent the percents of cases having each value.

Beginning of observation: In survival analysis, the moment in time when subjects begin to be followed by the researcher.

Between-subjects variable: A variable in repeated-measures ANOVA or linear mixed modeling that does not change over time for a given subject but takes on different values for different subjects.

Biased estimator: A sample statistic that is an inaccurate estimator of the corresponding population parameter; in particular, the mean of its sampling distribution is not equal to the population parameter.

Bivariate statistics: Statistical procedures for testing and assessing the association between two different variables.

Bonferroni post-hoc test: A multiple-comparison procedure allowing the researcher to test differences between pairs of group means without incurring capitalization on chance.

Capitalization on chance: The situation in which performing multiple tests of hypothesis raises the probability of rejecting a true null hypothesis beyond the alpha level desired for the group of tests.

Cases: The units of analysis in one's study. In logistic regression, however, the term also refers to the units of analysis who have experienced the event of interest.

Causal effect: The difference between the study endpoint's value if a subject experiences the treatment condition vs. its value if the same subject were to experience the control condition instead. This is a counterfactual definition because it is impossible to observe.

Censored cases: In survival analysis, these are cases with incompletely observed survival times. *Right censoring* occurs when the subject has not yet experienced the event by the end of the observation period. *Left censoring* occurs when subjects have already experienced the event by the beginning of observation.

Center of a distribution: The typical or average value in a variable's distribution.

Chi-squared (χ^2) test: A test of hypothesis used for testing the association between two qualitative variables or for testing model utility for models estimated with maximum likelihood.

Classification table: In logistic regression, a table showing the crosstabulation of a subject's actual status as case or control with the model's prediction of whether that subject is a case or control.

Clinical significance: The condition in which sample results that are significant are also clinically meaningful.

Confidence interval: An interval of numbers that we are very confident contains the true value of a population parameter.

Controls: In logistic regression, the units of analysis who have not experienced the event of interest.

Correlation coefficient: A measure ranging from -1 to $+1$ that indicates the strength and direction of linear association between two quantitative variables.

Cox regression model (a.k.a. proportional hazards model): The most commonly used regression model for survival data. The response variable is the log of the hazard function.

Crosstabulation (a.k.a. contingency) table: A table displaying the association between two qualitative variables.

Data: Numbers, letters, or special characters representing measurements of the properties of one's analytic units, or cases, in a study; data are the raw material of statistics.

Degrees of freedom: A technical term reflecting the number of independent elements comprising a statistical measure. Certain distributions require a degrees of freedom value to fully characterize them (e.g., the t, χ^2, and F distributions).

Descriptive statistics: The body of statistical techniques concerned with describing the salient features of the variables used in one's study.

Deviation score: The difference between a variable's value and the mean of the variable.

Directional conclusion: A conclusion in a two-tailed test that uses the nature of the sample results to suggest where the true parameter lies in relation to the null-hypothesized value.

Dispersion of a distribution: The degree of spread exhibited by a variable's values, typically assessed with the standard deviation.

Distribution (or probability distribution) of a variable: The collection of all values of a variable along with their associated probabilities of being observed.

Dummy variable: A variable in a regression model coded 1 if the case falls into a certain category of an explanatory variable and 0 otherwise. Used to represent qualitative predictors in a regression model.

Event count: The number of occurrences of an event to a subject within a given time period.

Experimental error: Random error that prevents study endpoints from being precisely determined by one or more explanatory variables.

Experimental study: Any study in which the study treatments (or levels of the explanatory variables) are randomly assigned to cases.

Explanatory variable (a.k.a. regressor, predictor, covariate): The causal variables in one's study that are used to explain the behavior of the study endpoint.

Exponential function: A mathematical operation in which Euler's constant (approximately equal to 2.72) is raised to the desired power.

External validity: The extent to which a study's results can be generalized to a larger, known population.

F test: A statistical test for which the null hypothesis is that all group means are the same (ANOVA) or that all regression coefficients equal zero in the population (linear regression).

False positive rate: In logistic regression, the probability of a control being mistakenly classified as a case by the prediction equation.

First quartile: The value in a distribution such that 25 % of the cases have lower values.

First-differenced estimator: An estimation method used in fixed-effects regression modeling that eliminates the fixed effect by using change scores for both the study endpoint and the explanatory variables.

Fixed effect: An unobserved characteristic of subjects that is both a predictor of the study endpoint and correlated with one or more explanatory variables in a regression model. Left unaddressed it will lead to biased regression estimates.

Fixed-effects regression model: A regression model in which the influence of unmeasured heterogeneity has been eliminated.

Growth-curve modeling (a.k.a. the linear mixed model): A regression analysis in which the response variable is the trajectory of change over time in a quantitative study endpoint. Interest centers on describing the average trajectory of change, as well as what subject characteristics lead to different trajectories of change for different types of subjects.

Hazard function: Approximately the instantaneous probability of experiencing the event of interest at any given time; this changes over time and is therefore a function of time.

Hazard ratio: The ratio of the hazard of event occurrence for subjects who are a unit apart on an explanatory variable.

Hosmer–Lemeshow test: A test of goodness-of-fit for a logistic regression model. It has a chi-squared distribution with eight degrees of freedom under the null hypothesis that the model fits. A significant value means the model does not fit the data well.

Hypothesis: A tentative statement about the value of one or more population parameters.

Ignorability of treatment assignment: The condition in which the potential outcomes of an experiment are independent of the manner in which treatment conditions are assigned to cases.

Inception of risk: In survival analysis, the moment in time when subjects come under the risk for an event.

Independent-samples, pooled-variance t test: A test for whether the means of two independently sampled groups are different; this test assumes that the variance of the study outcome is the same in each subpopulation.

Inferential statistics: The body of statistical techniques concerned with making inferences about a population based on drawing a sample from it.

Internal validity: The extent to which treatment-group differences on a study endpoint represent the causal effect of the treatment on the study endpoint.

Interquartile range (IQR): The difference between the first and third quartiles in a distribution.

Kaplan–Meier (a.k.a. product-limit) estimator: A nonparametric estimator of the survival function in survival analysis.

Left skewed: Said of distributions where most cases have high values of the variable, and a few outliers have very low values.

Left-truncated cases: Subjects in survival analysis who have already been at risk for event occurrence for some time when they come under observation.

Likelihood function: The formula for the probability of observing the collection of study endpoints observed in the sample, written as a function of the statistical model in question. Once a sample is collected, this formula is only influenced by the values of the coefficients in one's model.

Likelihood-ratio chi-squared test: The counterpart of linear regression's F test for logistic regression; this is a test of overall model utility.

Linear regression: A type of analysis in which a quantitative study endpoint is posited to be determined by one or more explanatory variables in a linear equation, i.e., a formula involving a weighted sum of coefficients times variables plus an error term.

Linearity in the parameters: The condition in which the right hand side of a statistical model is a weighted sum of coefficients times variables.

Log likelihood: The natural logarithm of the value of the likelihood function that is arrived at when coefficient estimates are plugged back into the likelihood function and the function is evaluated at those values. This property is not particularly informative but is nevertheless often reported when models are estimated via maximum likelihood.

Logistic regression: A regression model for the case in which the study endpoint is binary. The model holds that the log of the odds for the event in question is a linear function of the explanatory variables; estimation of the model is via maximum likelihood.

Logit transformation: The natural logarithm of the odds of the event.

Log-rank test: In survival analysis, a test for whether different groups of subjects have the same survival functions. An alternative test is the *Wilcoxon test*.

Maximum likelihood estimation: A means of estimating the coefficients of a statistical model that relies on finding the coefficient values that maximize the likelihood function for the collection of study endpoints in the sample.

Mean of a variable: The arithmetic average of the variable's values.

Mechanism: A characteristic that transmits the effect of one variable on another; also called an *intervening* variable or a *mediating* variable.

Median of a variable: The value of the variable such that half of the cases are lower in value and half are higher in value.

Missing at random: Said of missing data when the probability of being missing on a variable is unrelated to the value of that variable had it been observed.

Missing data: The problem of data being absent for one or more variables in one's study.

Mode: The most commonly occurring value in a distribution.

Multicollinearity: The situation in a regression model in which two are more predictors are highly correlated with each other, leading to poor-quality coefficient estimates.

Multinomial logistic regression: A logistic regression model for a study endpoint with more than two values.

Multiple imputation: A means of filling in missing data that involves using the interrelationships among variables in one's analysis, along with random error, to estimate the missing values. This process is repeated to create multiple copies of one's data; then one's statistical analysis of the data is repeated with each copy of the dataset and the results are combined into one final set of results.

Multiple-comparison procedure: A statistical procedure for comparing group means that avoids capitalization on chance.

Multivariate (or multivariable) analysis: An analysis in which one examines the simultaneous effect of two or more explanatory variables on a study endpoint.

Multivariate normal distribution: A multidimensional version of the normal distribution that characterizes a collection of variables. If a set of variables has a multivariate normal distribution, then the variables are all intercorrelated and each individual variable is normally distributed.

Natural logarithm: The number that Euler's constant (approximately 2.72) would be raised to in order to arrive at the value in question.

Negative binomial regression: Similar to Poisson regression except that there is no restriction that the mean and variance of the study endpoint must be identical.

Nonlinear association: An association between two quantitative variables in which the scatterplot does not follow a linear trend.

Nonlinear interaction effect: An interaction effect in which the nonlinear relationship between the study endpoint and an explanatory factor takes on different shapes over levels of another explanatory variable.

Nonlinear model: A statistical model that is not linear in the parameters, e.g., the logistic regression model, the Poisson regression model, the proportional hazards model.

Nonparametric test: A statistical test that makes very few assumptions about population distributions.

Nonprobability sample: A sample that is not a probability sample, i.e., a hand-picked sample, a convenience sample, a "snowball sample," etc. Study results using this type of sample can only be generalized to a hypothetical population.

Normal distribution: A population distribution that is symmetric and for which 68 % of cases are within one standard deviation of the mean, 95 % of cases are within two standard deviations of the mean, and approximately all cases are within three standard deviations of the mean. Certain sample statistics have a normal sampling distribution.

Null hypothesis: The opposite of the research hypothesis.

Observational study: Any study in which the study treatments (or levels of the explanatory variables) are not randomly assigned to cases.

Odds ratio: The ratio of the odds of an event for two different groups.

Odds: The ratio of probabilities for two different events for one group.

Offset: The log of the length of the time period over which an event count is taken, entered into a regression model with its coefficient constrained to equal 1. This converts the study endpoint into the rate of event occurrence.

One-tailed test: A test of hypothesis for which the research hypothesis is directional, i.e., if the null hypothesis is false, the true parameter value is hypothesized to be either strictly above the null-hypothesized value or strictly below it.

Ordinal logistic regression: A logistic regression model for a study endpoint with more than two values where the values also represent rank order on the characteristic of interest.

Ordinary least squares (a.k.a. OLS): A means of estimating coefficients in linear regression and ANOVA models that depends on finding the estimates that minimize the sum of squared prediction errors.

Orthogonality condition: The assumption that the experimental-error term in a statistical model is uncorrelated with the explanatory variables in the model.

Overdispersion parameter: A parameter in the negative binomial regression model that allows for the possibility that the variance of the study endpoint can be larger than the mean of the study endpoint.

P **value:** The probability of obtaining sample results as least as unfavorable to the null hypothesis as was observed if the null hypothesis is true.

Paired *t* test: A test for the difference between means for two groups when the groups are not independently sampled.

Parameter: A summary measure of some characteristic for the population, such as the population mean or proportion.

Partial likelihood estimation: The estimation method for the Cox regression model. It uses only the part of the likelihood function that is based exclusively on the regression coefficients.

Partial regression coefficient (a.k.a. partial slope): The coefficient for a predictor in a regression model that contains more than one explanatory variable. It represents the effect of that predictor controlling for all other predictors in the model.

Percentile: The value in a distribution such that a certain percentage of cases are lower than that value; for example, the 75th percentile is the value such that 75 % of cases have lower values.

Person-period data format: A type of dataset for statistical analysis in which each subject contributes to the dataset as many records as there are occasions on which that subject was measured. Datasets in this format are often necessary in survival analysis and growth-curve analysis.

Poisson distribution: A probability distribution for an integer variable representing an event count.

Poisson regression: A type of regression analysis in which the study endpoint is a count of the number of occurrences of an event that has happened to subjects in some fixed period of time.

Population: The total collection of cases the researcher wishes to generalize the results of his or her study to.

Power of the test: The probability that one will reject a false null hypothesis with a particular statistical test.

Predictive nomogram: A mathematical formula, based on statistical modeling, which facilitates forecasting patient outcomes. In survival analysis, the predicted outcome is typically the probability of surviving a given length of time before experiencing the study endpoint.

Probability sample: A type of sample for which one can specify the probability that any member of the population will be selected into it. This type of sample enables generalization of the study results to a known population.

Propensity scores: Predicted probabilities of receiving the treatment for different subjects. Subjects who have the same propensity scores can be treated in statistical analyses as though they were randomly assigned to treatment groups.

Propensity-score analysis: Any statistical analysis that controls for propensity scores and thereby balances the distributions on control variables across groups of subjects.

Pseudo-R^2 measure: Any of several analogs of the linear regression R^2 used for nonlinear models such as logistic regression, Poisson regression, Cox regression, etc.

Quadratic model: A regression model that includes a variable along with its square as explanatory factors in the model. Such a model allows for a nonlinear relationship between the study endpoint and that factor; the curve describing that relationship would be able to have one bend in it.

Qualitative variable: A variable whose values indicate a difference in kind, or nature, only. Even if represented by numbers (which they usually are), the values convey no quantitative meaning.

Quantitative variable: A variable whose values indicate either the exact amount of the characteristic present or a rank order on the characteristic.

R^2: A measure of the strength of association between a quantitative study endpoint and one or more quantitative explanatory variables. It has the additional property that it can be interpreted as the proportion of variation in the study endpoint that is accounted for by the explanatory variable(s).

Range: The difference between the highest and lowest values in a distribution.

Rate of event occurrence: An event count divided by the time period over which the count is taken.

Receiver operating characteristic (ROC) curve: In logistic regression, a curve showing the sensitivity of classification plotted against the false positive rate as the criterion probability is varied from 0 to 1. Used to indicate the predictive efficacy, or discriminatory power, of the model.

Relative risk: The ratio of the probability of an event for two different groups.

Repeated-measures ANOVA: A type of ANOVA in which subjects are repeatedly measured on the study endpoint over time, so that time becomes an additional explanatory variable in the analysis. Often repeated-measures ANOVA features a treatment factor and time as the two explanatory variables.

Research hypothesis: The hypothesis that the researcher is trying to marshal evidence for; this is usually the hypothesis that is suggested either by prior research or theory as being true.

Reverse causation: The situation in which the study endpoint in a regression model is actually the cause of one of the explanatory variables in the model, rather than the other way around.

Right skewed: Said of distributions where most cases have low values of the variable, and a few outliers have very high values.

Risk set: In survival analysis, the total group of subjects who are at risk for event occurrence at any given time.

Robust: The property of a statistical procedure of providing valid results even when the assumptions for that procedure are not met.

Sampling distribution: The probability distribution for a sample statistic; this distribution determines the p values for statistical tests.

Sampling to a population: Conjuring up a hypothetical population that nonprobability sample results might be generalizable to by imagining repeating the sampling procedure ad infinitum to generate a population. One's current sample can then be considered a random sample from this hypothetical population.

Scatterplot: A graphical display of the association between two quantitative variables achieved by plotting points representing the intersection of each variable's values.

Selection bias: Bias in one's regression estimates brought about either by an unmeasured characteristic of cases that causes only certain kinds of cases to be assigned certain treatments (*self-selection bias*) or by an unmeasured characteristic that causes only certain kinds of cases to be present in one's sample (*sample-selection bias*).

Sensitivity analysis: An alternative analysis using a different model or different assumptions to explore whether one's main findings are robust to different analytical approaches to the research problem.

Sensitivity of classification: In logistic regression, the probability of a case being classified as a case by the prediction equation.

Simple random sample: A sample in which every member of the population has the same chance of being selected into the sample.

Specificity of classification: In logistic regression, the probability of a control being classified as a control by the prediction equation.

Standard deviation: The square root of a variable's variance. The standard deviation is the most commonly used measure of dispersion, and represents approximately the average distance of values from the mean of a distribution.

Standard error: The standard deviation of the sampling distribution of a statistic.

Statistical control: Statistically holding other explanatory variables constant when looking at the effect of a given predictor on a study endpoint. It is designed to mimic the kind of control achieved with random assignment to levels of the predictor. However, it is no substitute for random assignment, as it only controls for *measured* characteristics.

Statistical interaction (a.k.a. stratification effects): The situation in which the nature of the association between a predictor and a study endpoint is different for different levels of a third variable.

Statistical model: A set of one or more equations describing the process or processes that generated the scores on the study endpoint.

Statistical significance: The condition in which the p value for a statistical test is below the alpha level for the test, leading to rejection of the null hypothesis.

Strength of association: The degree to which knowledge of one's status on one variable enables prediction of one's status on another variable that it is associated with. Measures of strength of association ideally range in absolute value from 0 to 1.

Study endpoint (a.k.a. outcome, dependent variable, criterion variable or response variable): The "effect" variable whose "behavior" one is trying to explain using one or more explanatory variables in the study.

Subclassification on propensity scores: A means of performing propensity-score analysis in which the substantive analysis is repeated on different groups having roughly the same propensity scores. The analysis results from the different groups are then combined into one final result via weighted averaging.

Survival analysis: The analysis of time-to-event data, i.e., the length of time until an event occurs to subjects. The most popular multivariable technique, Cox regression, is a model for the log of the hazard of the event.

Survival function: The probability of surviving to a particular point in time without experiencing the event of interest; this changes over time and is therefore a function of time.

Symmetric: Said of distributions that exhibit no skewness, and for which exactly 50 % of cases lie above and below the mean of the distribution.

T **distribution:** A population distribution that is symmetric and resembles the normal distribution except that it exhibits more dispersion. Some sample statistics have a *t* sampling distribution.

Test of hypothesis: A statistical test of the plausibility of the null hypothesis in a study.

Test statistic: A sample statistic measuring the discrepancy between what is observed in the sample, as opposed to what one would expect to observe if the null hypothesis were true. A requirement for a test statistic is that it must have a known sampling distribution if the null hypothesis is true.

The central limit theorem: A mathematical theorem specifying the sampling distribution of a sample statistic (e.g., the sample mean) when the researcher has a large sample.

Third quartile: The value in a distribution such that 75 % of cases have lower values.

Time-varying covariates: Explanatory variables whose values can change at different occasions of measurement for the same subject.

Two-tailed test: A test of hypothesis for which the research hypothesis is not directional, i.e., the research hypothesis allows for the possibility that the true parameter value could fall on either side of the null-hypothesized value.

Type I error: The probability of rejecting a true null hypothesis in a statistical test.

Type II error: The probability of failing to reject a false null hypothesis in a statistical test.

Unbiased estimator: A sample statistic for which the mean of its sampling distribution is equal to the population parameter it is designed to estimate; this is considered a desirable property of an estimator.

Uncensored cases: In survival analysis, those subjects who experience the event of interest during the observation period of the study.

Unmeasured heterogeneity: An unmeasured characteristic of one's cases that is related to one or more explanatory variables in the study, as well as the study endpoint. Part or all of the supposed "effect" of the explanatory variables on the study endpoint is actually attributable to this unmeasured confounding factor.

Variance of a variable: The average of the squared deviation scores.

Wilcoxon rank sum test: A nonparametric test for the difference in the study endpoint between two independently sampled groups.

Within-subjects variable: A variable in repeated-measures ANOVA or linear mixed modeling that takes on different values over time for the same subject.

Φ^2: A measure of the strength of association for two qualitative variables that are each binary variables. It is equivalent to the square of the correlation coefficient for quantitative variables.

References

Abouassaly, R., Alibhai, S. M. H., Tomlinson, G. A., Urbach, D. R., & Finelli, A. (2011). The effect of age on the morbidity of kidney surgery. *The Journal of Urology, 186*, 811–816.

Agresti, A. (1990). *Categorical data analysis*. New York: Wiley.

Agresti, A., & Finlay, B. (2009). *Statistical methods for the social sciences* (4th ed.). Upper Saddle River, NJ: Prentice Hall.

Allison, P. D. (1982). Discrete-time methods for the analysis of event histories. In S. Leinhardt (Ed.), *Sociological Methodology 1982* (pp. 61–98). San Francisco: Jossey-Bass.

Allison, P. D. (2002). *Missing data*. Thousand Oaks, CA: Sage.

Allison, P. D. (2005). *Fixed effects regression methods for longitudinal data using SAS*. Cary, NC: SAS Institute Inc.

Allison, P. D. (2009). *Fixed effects regression models*. Thousand Oaks, CA: Sage.

Allison, P. D. (2010). *Survival analysis using SAS: A practical guide* (2nd ed.). Cary, NC: SAS Institute Inc.

Anton, H. (1984). *Calculus* (2nd ed.). New York: Wiley.

Antonarakis, E. S., Feng, Z., Trock, B. J., Humphreys, E. B., Carducci, M. A., Partin, A. W., et al. (2011). The natural history of metastatic progression in men with prostate-specific antigen recurrence after radical prostatectomy: Long-term follow-up. *BJU International, 109*, 32–39.

Bendavid, E., Holmes, C. B., Bhattacharya, J., & Miller, G. (2012). HIV development assistance and adult mortality in Africa. *Journal of the American Medical Association, 307*, 2060–2067.

Bien, T. H., Miller, W. R., & Tonigan, J. S. (1993). Brief interventions for alcohol problems: a review. *Addiction, 88*, 315–335.

Bollen, K. A. (1989). *Structural equations with latent variables*. New York: Wiley.

Cameron, A. C., & Trivedi, P. K. (1998). *Regression analysis of count data*. Cambridge, UK: Cambridge University Press.

Capitanio, U., Suardi, N., Briganti, A., Gallina, A., Abdollah, Lughezzani, G., et al. (2011). Influence of obesity on tumour volume in patients with prostate cancer. *BJU International, 109*, 678–684.

Cobain, K., Owens, L., Ruwanthi, K., Fitzgerald, R., Gilmore, I., & Pirmohamed, M. (2011). Brief interventions in dependent drinkers: A comparative prospective analysis in two hospitals. *Alcohol and Alcoholism, 46*, 434–440.

Crawford, E. D., Moul, J. W., Rove, K. O., Pettaway, C. A., Lamerato, L. E., & Hughes, A. (2011). Prostate-specific antigen 1.5–4.0 ng/mL: A diagnostic challenge and danger zone. *BJU International, 108*, 1743–1749.

DeMaris, A. (2002). Explained variance in logistic regression: A Monte Carlo study of proposed measures. *Sociological Methods & Research, 31*, 27–74.

A. DeMaris and S.H. Selman, *Converting Data into Evidence: A Statistics Primer for the Medical Practitioner*, DOI 10.1007/978-1-4614-7792-1,
© Springer Science+Business Media New York 2013

DeMaris, A. (2004). *Regression with social data: Modeling continuous and limited response variables*. Hoboken, NJ: Wiley.

DeMaris, A. (2012). *Combating self-selection bias in nonexperimental research: A Monte Carlo Study*. Manuscript submitted for publication.

DeMaris, A. (2013). Logistic regression: Basic foundations and new directions. In I. B. Weiner (Series Ed.), W. Velicer, & J. Schinka (Vol. Eds.), *Handbook of Psychology: Vol. 2. Research methods in psychology* (2nd ed., pp. 543–570). Hoboken, NJ: Wiley.

DeMaris, A., Mahoney, A., & Pargament, K. I. (2010). Sanctification of marriage and general religiousness as buffers of the effects of marital inequity. *Journal of Family issues, 31*, 1255–1278.

DeMaris, A., Mahoney, A., & Pargament, K. I. (2011). Doing the scut work of infant care: Does religiousness encourage father involvement? *Journal of Marriage and Family, 73*, 354–368.

Duncan, B., & Rees, D. I. (2005). Effect of smoking on depressive symptomatology: A reexamination of data from the National Longitudinal Study of Adolescent Health. *American Journal of Epidemiology, 162*, 461–470.

Emara, A. M., Chadwick, E., Nobes, J. P., Abdelbaky, A. M., Laing, R. W., & Langley, S. E. M. (2011). Long-term toxicity and quality of life up to 10 years after low-does rate brachytherapy for prostate cancer. *BJU International, 109*, 994–1000.

Fitzmaurice, G. M., Laird, N. M., & Ware, J. H. (2004). *Applied longitudinal analysis*. Hoboken, NJ: Wiley.

Flensner, G., Ek, A., Soderhamn, O., & Landtblom, A. (2011). Sensitivity to heat in MS patients: A factor strongly influencing symptomology – an explorative survey. *BMC Neurology, 11*:27.

Gill, J. (2001). *Generalized linear models: A unified approach*. Thousand Oaks, CA: Sage.

Ginting, J. V., Tripp, D. A., Nickel, C., Fitzgerald, M. P., & Mayer, R. (2010). Spousal support decreases the negative impact of pain on mental quality of life in women with interstitial cystitis/painful bladder syndrome. *BJU International, 108*, 713–717.

Green, R. C., Schneider, L. S., Amato, D., Beelen, A. P., Wilcock, G., Swabb, E. A., et al. (2009). Effect of tarenflurbil on cognitive decline and activities of daily living in patients with mild Alzheimer disease. *Journal of the American Medical Association, 302*, 2557–2564.

Guo, S., & Fraser, M. W. (2010). *Propensity score analysis: Statistical methods and applications*. Thousand Oaks, CA: Sage.

Guyatt, G. H. (1991). Evidence based medicine. *American College of Physicians Journal Club, 114*, A16.

Harrell, F. E., Jr., Lee, K. L., & Mark, D. B. (1996). Multivariable prognostic models: Issues in developing models, evaluating assumptions and adequacy, and measuring and reducing errors. *Statistics in Medicine, 15*, 361–387.

Hewitt, B., & Turrell, G. (2011). Short-term functional health and well-being after marital separation: Does initiator status make a difference? *American Journal of Epidemiology, 173*, 1308–1318.

Ho, C. C. K., Tong, S. F., Low, W. Y., Ng, C. J., Khoo, E. M., Lee, V. K. M., et al. (2011). A randomized, double-blind, placebo-controlled trial on the effect of long-acting testosterone treatment as assessed by the Aging Male Symptoms scale. *BJU International, 110*, 260–265.

Hosmer, D. W., & Lemeshow, S. (1999). *Applied survival analysis: Regression modeling of time to event data*. New York: Wiley.

Hosmer, D. W., & Lemeshow, S. (2000). *Applied logistic regression* (2nd ed.). New York: Wiley.

Hunte, H. E. R. (2011). Association between perceived interpersonal everyday discrimination and waist circumference over a 9-year period in the Midlife Development in the United States Cohort Study. *American Journal of Epidemiology, 173*, 1232–1239.

Jagsi, R., Griffith, K. A., Stewart, A., Sambuco, D., DeCastro, R., & Ubel, P. A. (2012). Gender differences in the salaries of physician researchers. *Journal of the American Medical Association, 307*, 2410–2417.

Johnson, D. R., & Young, R. (2011). Toward best practices in analyzing datasets with missing data: Comparisons and recommendations. *Journal of Marriage and Family, 73*, 926–945.

Jung, H., Kim, K. H., Yoon, S. J., & Kim, T. B. (2010). Second to fourth digit ratio: A predictor of prostate-specific antigen level and the presence of prostate cancer. *BJU International, 107*, 591–596.

Khawaja, O., Kotler, G., Gaziano, J. M., & Djousse, L. (2012). Usefulness of desirable lifestyle factors to attenuate the risk of heart failure among offspring whose parents had myocardial infarction before age 55 years. *American Journal of Cardiology, 110*, 326–330.

King, G. (1988). Statistical models for political science event counts: Bias in conventional procedures and evidence for the exponential Poisson regression model. *American Journal of Political Science, 32*, 838–863.

Li, R., Louie, M. K., Lee, H. J., Osann, K., Pick, D. L., Santos, R., et al. (2010). Prospective randomized trial of three different methods of nephrostomy tract closure after percutaneous nephrolithotripsy. *BJU International, 107*, 1660–1665.

Lieb, W., Beiser, A. S., Ramachandran, S. V., Tan, Z. S., Au, R., Harris, T. B., et al. (2009). Association of plasma leptin levels with incident Alzheimer disease and MRI measures of brain aging. *Journal of the American Medical Association, 302*, 2565–2572.

Little, R. J. A., & Rubin, D. B. (1987). *Statistical analysis with missing data.* New York: Wiley.

Liu, R., Guo, X., Park, Y., Huang, X., Sinha, R., Freedman, N. D., et al. (2012). Caffeine intake, smoking, and risk of Parkinson disease in men and women. *American Journal of Epidemiology, 175*, 1200–1207.

Long, J. S. (1997). *Regression models for categorical and limited dependent variables.* Thousand Oaks, CA: Sage.

Mahoney, A., Pargament, K. I., & DeMaris, A. (2009). Couples viewing marriage and pregnancy through the lens of the sacred: A descriptive study. *Research in the Social Scientific Study of Religion, 20*, 1–45.

Marcus, S. M., Stuart, E. A., Wang, P., Shadish, W. R., & Steiner, P. M. (2012). Estimating the causal effect of randomization versus treatment preference in a doubly randomized preference trial. *Psychological Methods, 17*, 244–254.

Mirowsky, J., & Ross, C. E. (1984). Components of depressed mood in married men and women: The Center for Epidemiological Studies depression scale. *American Journal of Epidemiology, 119*, 997–1004.

Moayyedi, P. (2008). CON: Evidence-based medicine—the emperor's new clothes? *American Journal of Gastroenterology 103*, 2967–2969.

Morgan, T. M., Keegan, K. A., Barocas, D. A., Ruhotina, N. Phillips, S. E., Chang, S. S., et al. (2011). Predicting the probability of 90-day survival of elderly patients with bladder cancer treated with radical cystectomy. *The Journal of Urology, 186*, 829–834.

Motl, R. W., Suh, Y., Balantrapu, S., Sandroff, B., Sosnoff, J. J., Pula, J., et al. (2012). Evidence for the different physiological significance of the 6- and 2-minute walk tests in multiple sclerosis. *BMC Neurology, 12*:6

Nickel, J. C., Gilling, P., Tammela, T. L., Morrill, B. Wilson, T. H., & Rittmaster, R. S. (2011). Comparison of dutasteride and finasteride for treating benign prostatic hyperplasia: The Enlarged Prostate International Comparator Study (EPICS). *BJU International, 108*, 388–394.

O'Brien, B. A., Cohen, R. J., Wheeler, T. M., & Moorin, R. E. (2010). A post-radical-prostatectomy nomogram incorporating new pathological variables and interaction terms for improved prognosis. *BJU International, 107*, 389–395.

Ott, L. (1988). *An introduction to statistical methods and data analysis.* Boston: PWS-Kent.

Paton, N. I., Goodall, R. L., Dunn, D. T., Franzen, S., Collaco-Moraes, Y., Gazzard, B. G., et al. (2012). Effects of hydroxychloroquine on immune activation and disease progression among HIV-infected patients not receiving antiretroviral therapy: A randomized controlled trial. *Journal of the American Medical Association, 308*, 353–361.

Pettaway, C. A., Lamerato, L. E., Eaddy, M. T., Edwards, J. K., Hogue, S. L., & Crane, M. M. (2011). Benign prostatic hyperplasia: Racial differences in treatment patterns and prostate cancer prevalence. *BJU International, 108*, 1302–1308.

Ranasinghe, W. K. B., Wright, T., Attia, J., McElduff, P., Doyle, T., Bartholomew, M., et al. (2010). Effects of bariatric surgery on urinary and sexual function. *BJU International, 107*, 88–94.

Raudenbush, S. W., & Bryk, A. S. (2002). *Hierarchical linear models: Applications and data analysis methods* (2nd ed.). Thousand Oaks, CA: Sage.

Rosenfeld, M., Ratjen, F., Brumback, L., Daniel, S., Rowbotham, R., McNamara, S., et al. (2012). Inhaled hypertonic saline in infants and children younger than 6 years with cystic fibrosis: The ISIS randomized controlled trial. *Journal of the American Medical Association, 307*, 2269–2277.

Rubin, D. B. (2001). Using propensity scores to help design observational studies: Application to the tobacco litigation. *Health Services and Outcomes Research Methodology, 2*, 169–188.

Schafer, J. L. (2000). *Analysis of incomplete multivariate data.* Boca Raton, FL: Chapman & Hall/CRC.

Schafer, J. L., & Kang, J. (2008). Average causal effects from nonrandomized studies: A practical guide and simulated example. *Psychological Methods, 13*, 279–313.

Singer, J. D., & Willett, J. B. (2003) *Applied longitudinal data analysis: Modeling change and event occurrence.* New York: Oxford University Press.

Singleton, R. A., Jr., & Straits, B. C. (2010). *Approaches to social research.* New York: Oxford University Press.

Subramanian, S., Tawakol, A., Burdo, T. H., Abbara, S., Wei, J., Vijayakumar, J., et al. (2012). Arterial inflammation in patients with HIV. *Journal of the American Medical Association, 308*, 379–386.

Tynjala, J., Kangastupa, P., Laatikainen, T., Aalto, M., & Niemela, O. (2012). Effect of age and gender on the relationship between alcohol consumption and serum GGT: Time to recalibrate goals for normal ranges. *Alcohol and Alcoholism, 47*, 558–562.

Umberson, D., Liu, H., & Powers, D. (2009). Marital status, marital transitions, and body weight. *Journal of Health and Social Behavior, 50*, 327–343.

Wahbi, K., Meune, C., Porcher, R., Becane, H. M., Lazarus, A., Laforet, P., et al. (2012). Electrophysiolgical study with prophylactic pacing and survival in adults with myotonic dystrophy and conduction system disease. *Journal of the American Medical Association, 307*, 1292–1301.

West, S. G., & Thoemmes, F. (2010). Campbell's and Rubin's perspectives on causal inference. *Psychological Methods, 15*, 18–37.

Wilhelm-Leen, E. R., Hall, Y. N., deBoer, I. H., & Chertow, G. M. (2010). Vitamin D deficiency and frailty in older Americans. *Journal of Internal Medicine, 268*, 171–180.

Wooldridge, J. M. (2002). *Econometric analysis of cross section and panel data.* Cambridge, MA: MIT Press.

Yafi, F. A., Aprikian, A. G., Chin, J. L., Fradet, Y., Izawa, J., Estey, E., et al. (2010). Contemporary outcomes of 2287 patients with bladder cancer who were treated with radical cystectomy: A Canadian multicentre experience. *BJU International, 108*, 539–545.

Yu, H., Hevelone, N. D., Lipsitz, S. R., Kowalczyk, K. J., Nguyen, P. L., & Hu, J. C. (2012). Hospital volume, utilization costs and outcomes of robot-assisted laparoscopic radical prostatectomy. *The Journal of Urology, 187*, 1632–1638.

Zolna, M. R., & Lindberg, L. D. (2012). *Unintended pregnancy: Incidence and outcomes among young adult unmarried women in the United States, 2001 and 2008.* New York: Guttmacher Institute.

About the Authors

Alfred DeMaris earned a Ph.D. in sociology from the University of Florida in 1982 and a master's degree in statistics from Virginia Tech in 1987. He is currently professor of sociology and statistician for the Center for Family and Demographic Research at Bowling Green State University in Bowling Green, Ohio. His other statistical monographs are *Logit Modeling: Practical Applications* (Sage, 1992) and *Regression with Social Data: Modeling Continuous and Limited Response Variables* (Wiley, 2004). He has published another dozen articles and book chapters on statistical techniques as well as approximately 70 journal articles on topics in family social psychology. His work has appeared in *Psychological Bulletin, Sociological Methods & Research, Social Forces, Social Psychology Quarterly, Journal of Marriage and Family*, and *Journal of Family Issues*, among other venues. He was twice awarded the Hugo Beigel Award for the best empirical article in the *Journal of Sex Research*. He has been teaching statistics at the undergraduate and graduate levels for the past 30 years. Through his company, Statistical Insights, he does statistical consulting on a regular basis for individuals in the social and behavioral sciences as well as those in medicine and industry.

Steven Selman received his undergraduate degree in Engineering Physics at the University of Toledo. Following his medical school training at Case Western Reserve University, he completed residencies both in General Surgery and Urology at University Hospitals of Cleveland. His research interest has principally been in the arena of urologic oncology and methodologies of urologic resident education. He has over 100 publications in the peer-reviewed urologic literature. Currently, Dr. Selman serves both as residency Program Director and Chair of the Department of Urology at University of Toledo Medical Center.

A. DeMaris and S.H. Selman, *Converting Data into Evidence: A Statistics Primer for the Medical Practitioner*, DOI 10.1007/978-1-4614-7792-1,
© Springer Science+Business Media New York 2013

Index

A. DeMaris and S.H. Selman, *Converting Data into Evidence: A Statistics Primer*
for the Medical Practitioner, DOI 10.1007/978-1-4614-7792-1,
© Springer Science+Business Media New York 2013

Lightning Source UK Ltd.
Milton Keynes UK
UKOW06f1818040615

252893UK00003B/6/P